Chagas Disease

Chagas Disease

Editors

Jorg Heukelbach
Alberto Novaes Ramos Jr.
Andréa Silvestre de Sousa

MDPI • Basel • Beijing • Wuhan • Barcelona • Belgrade • Manchester • Tokyo • Cluj • Tianjin

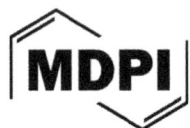

Editors
Jorg Heukelbach
Federal University of Ceará
Brazil

Alberto Novaes Ramos Jr.
Federal University of Ceará
Brazil

Andréa Silvestre de Sousa
Evandro Chagas National Institute of Infectious Diseases
Brazil

Editorial Office
MDPI
St. Alban-Anlage 66
4052 Basel, Switzerland

This is a reprint of articles from the Special Issue published online in the open access journal *Tropical Medicine and Infectious Disease* (ISSN 2414-6366) (available at: https://www.mdpi.com/journal/tropicalmed/special_issues/chagas_disease).

For citation purposes, cite each article independently as indicated on the article page online and as indicated below:

LastName, A.A.; LastName, B.B.; LastName, C.C. Article Title. *Journal Name* **Year**, *Volume Number*, Page Range.

ISBN 978-3-0365-1248-8 (Hbk)
ISBN 978-3-0365-1249-5 (PDF)

Cover image courtesy of Collection of Casa de Oswaldo Cruz/Fiocruz, Rio de Janeiro, Brazil.

© 2021 by the authors. Articles in this book are Open Access and distributed under the Creative Commons Attribution (CC BY) license, which allows users to download, copy and build upon published articles, as long as the author and publisher are properly credited, which ensures maximum dissemination and a wider impact of our publications.

The book as a whole is distributed by MDPI under the terms and conditions of the Creative Commons license CC BY-NC-ND.

Contents

About the Editors vii

Jorg Heukelbach, Andréa Silvestre de Sousa and Alberto Novaes Ramos Jr.
New Contributions to the Elimination of Chagas Disease as a Public Health Problem: Towards the Sustainable Development Goals by 2030
Reprinted from: *Trop. Med. Infect. Dis.* **2021**, *6*, 23, doi:10.3390/tropicalmed6010023 1

Simone Petraglia Kropf and Nísia Trindade Lima
The 14th of April, Past and Present
Reprinted from: *Trop. Med. Infect. Dis.* **2020**, *5*, 100, doi:10.3390/tropicalmed5020100 5

Mario J Olivera, Francisco Palencia-Sánchez and Martha Riaño-Casallas
The Cost of Lost Productivity Due to Premature Chagas Disease-Related Mortality: Lessons from Colombia (2010–2017)
Reprinted from: *Trop. Med. Infect. Dis.* **2021**, *6*, 17, doi:10.3390/tropicalmed6010017 9

Liliane da Rocha Siriano, Andrea Marchiol, Marina Pereira Certo, Juan-Carlos Cubides, Colin Forsyth and Fabrício Augusto de Sousa
Mandatory Notification of Chronic Chagas Disease: Confronting the Epidemiological Silence in the State of Goiás, Brazil
Reprinted from: *Trop. Med. Infect. Dis.* **2020**, *5*, 92, doi:10.3390/tropicalmed5020092 17

Ana Yecê das Neves Pinto, Vera da Costa Valente, Sebastião Aldo da Silva Valente, Tamires Anastácia Rodrigues Motta and Ana Maria Revorêdo da Silva Ventura
Clinical, Cardiological and Serologic Follow-Up of Chagas Disease in Children and Adolescents from the Amazon Region, Brazil: Longitudinal Study
Reprinted from: *Trop. Med. Infect. Dis.* **2020**, *5*, 139, doi:10.3390/tropicalmed5030139 27

Alejandro Marcel Hasslocher-Moreno, Sergio Salles Xavier, Roberto Magalhães Saraiva, Luiz Henrique Conde Sangenis, Marcelo Teixeira de Holanda, Henrique Horta Veloso, Andrea Rodrigues da Costa, Fernanda de Souza Nogueira Sardinha Mendes, Pedro Emmanuel Alvarenga Americano do Brasil, Gilberto Marcelo Sperandio da Silva, Mauro Felippe Felix Mediano and Andrea Silvestre de Sousa
Progression Rate from the Indeterminate Form to the Cardiac Form in Patients with Chronic Chagas Disease: Twenty-Two-Year Follow-Up in a Brazilian Urban Cohort
Reprinted from: *Trop. Med. Infect. Dis.* **2020**, *5*, 76, doi:10.3390/tropicalmed5020076 39

Joao Manoel Rossi Neto, Marco Aurelio Finger and Carolina Casadei dos Santos
Benznidazole as Prophylaxis for Chagas Disease Infection Reactivation in Heart Transplant Patients: A Case Series in Brazil
Reprinted from: *Trop. Med. Infect. Dis.* **2020**, *5*, 132, doi:10.3390/tropicalmed5030132 51

Leandro S. Sangenito, Marta H. Branquinha and André L. S. Santos
Funding for Chagas Disease: A 10-Year (2009–2018) Survey
Reprinted from: *Trop. Med. Infect. Dis.* **2020**, *5*, 88, doi:10.3390/tropicalmed5020088 57

Aaron W. Tustin, Ricardo Castillo-Neyra, Laura D. Tamayo, Renzo Salazar, Katty Borini-Mayorí and Michael Z. Levy
Elucidating the Mechanism of *Trypanosoma cruzi* Acquisition by Triatomine Insects: Evidence from a Large Field Survey of *Triatoma infestans*
Reprinted from: *Trop. Med. Infect. Dis.* **2020**, *5*, 87, doi:10.3390/tropicalmed5020087 69

Fernando Mussa Abujamra Aith, Colin Forsyth and Maria Aparecida Shikanai-Yasuda
Chagas Disease and Healthcare Rights in the Bolivian Immigrant Community of São Paulo, Brazil
Reprinted from: *Trop. Med. Infect. Dis.* **2020**, *5*, 62, doi:10.3390/tropicalmed5020062 . . . . **79**

Jose Luis Ramirez
Trypanosoma cruzi Genome 15 Years Later: What Has Been Accomplished?
Reprinted from: *Trop. Med. Infect. Dis.* **2020**, *5*, 129, doi:10.3390/tropicalmed5030129 . . . . **91**

Maria da Consolação Vieira Moreira and José Renan Cunha-Melo
Chagas Disease Infection Reactivation after Heart Transplant
Reprinted from: *Trop. Med. Infect. Dis.* **2020**, *5*, 106, doi:10.3390/tropicalmed5030106 . . . . **101**

Renata J. Moll-Bernardes, Paulo Henrique Rosado-de-Castro, Gabriel Cordeiro Camargo, Fernanda Souza Nogueira Sardinha Mendes, Adriana S. X. Brito and Andréa Silvestre Sousa
New Imaging Parameters to Predict Sudden Cardiac Death in Chagas Disease
Reprinted from: *Trop. Med. Infect. Dis.* **2020**, *5*, 74, doi:10.3390/tropicalmed5020074 . . . . **113**

Fernanda de Souza Nogueira Sardinha Mendes, Mauro Felippe Felix Mediano, Rudson Santos Silva, Sergio Salles Xavier, Pedro Emmanuel Alvarenga Americano do Brasil, Roberto Magalhães Saraiva, Alejandro Marcel Hasslocher-Moreno and Andrea Silvestre de Sousa
Discussing the Score of Cardioembolic Ischemic Stroke in Chagas Disease
Reprinted from: *Trop. Med. Infect. Dis.* **2020**, *5*, 82, doi:10.3390/tropicalmed5020082 . . . . **125**

Karine Rezende-Oliveira, Cesar Gómez-Hernández, Marcos Vinícius da Silva, Rafael Faria de Oliveira, Juliana Reis Machado, Luciana de Almeida Silva Teixeira, Lúcio Roberto Cançado Castellano, Dalmo Correia and Virmondes Rodrigues
Effects of Meglumine Antimoniate Treatment on Cytokine Production in a Patient with Mucosal Leishmaniasis and Chagas Diseases Co-Infection
Reprinted from: *Trop. Med. Infect. Dis.* **2020**, *5*, 69, doi:10.3390/tropicalmed5020069 . . . . **131**

About the Editors

Jorg Heukelbach, MD MScIH Ph.D., is an internationally renowned specialist in the area of epidemiology and control of neglected tropical diseases and One Health, with extensive experience in many countries worldwide. He is a Professor at the Federal University of Ceará (Brazil) and Editor-in-Chief of the journal *One Health and Implementation Research*.

Alberto Novaes Ramos Jr. MD MPH Ph.D., is a Professor of Epidemiology and Research Methods in Public Health at the School of Medicine of the Federal University of Ceará, Northeast Brazil. He graduated in Medicine from the Federal University of Rio de Janeiro (UFRJ) in 1996, and concluded his specialization in Infectious and Parasitic Diseases (UFRJ) and in Family and Community Medicine. He leads a research group focused on tropical medicine, public health, and infectious disease epidemiology (with an emphasis on Chagas disease, leprosy, schistosomiasis, leishmaniasis, syphilis, and HIV/AIDS) and health research methodology (health systems research, implementation research, and operational research). He participated as a member of Technical Advisory Committees of the Brazilian Ministry of Health (STI/AIDS, Leprosy, Chagas Disease, Neglected Tropical Diseases, Hemovigilance and Development of Operational Research, among others). He was part of the technical coordination group of the first (2005) and the second (2015) Brazilian Consensus on Chagas Disease. He was a member and coordinator of the Brazilian Attention and Studies Network on Co-Infection *Trypanosoma cruzi* and HIV. He is Associate Editor of *Cadernos de Saúde Pública/Reports in Public Health* (ENSP-Fiocruz), *Cadernos Saúde Coletiv*a (IESC-UFRJ), *Revista Brasileira de Medicina de Família e Comunidade/Brazilian Journal of Family and Community Medicine* (SBMFC), and *PLoS Neglected Tropical Diseases* (PLoS). In all projects, social and environmental determinants of health, vulnerabilities, and health inequalities are included. He has actively participated in Brazilian and international campaigns against Neglected Tropical Diseases with a focus on Chagas disease, empowerment, and human rights.

Andréa Silvestre de Sousa, MD Ph.D., is a Researcher at the National Institute of Infectious Diseases Evandro Chagas (INI) of the Oswaldo Cruz Foundation (Fiocruz) and Adjunct Professor of Cardiology at the School of Medicine of Federal University of Rio de Janeiro (UFRJ). Graduated in Medicine at the UFRJ in 1995, she concluded her specialization in Cardiology (UFRJ) in 1998. She started her research activity in 1999 at the Department of Clinical Medicine at the Federal University of Rio de Janeiro, where she obtained her Master's degree (2000) and a PhD (2003) in Medicine (Cardiology). Since 2018, she has been the Head of the Clinical Research Laboratory for Chagas disease at INI-Fiocruz. She has experience in the field of Medicine, with an emphasis on Cardiology, working mainly on the following topics: Chagas disease, chronic Chagas heart disease, heart failure, cardiac rehabilitation, and echocardiography. She worked in different epidemiological scenarios as a doctor and researcher in Chagas disease, working with a strong interface with primary health care.

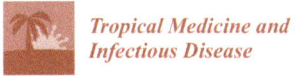

Editorial

New Contributions to the Elimination of Chagas Disease as a Public Health Problem: Towards the Sustainable Development Goals by 2030

Jorg Heukelbach [1,*], Andréa Silvestre de Sousa [2] and Alberto Novaes Ramos Jr. [1,3]

1. Postgraduate Course in Public Health, School of Medicine, Federal University of Ceará, Fortaleza, CE 60430-140, Brazil; novaes@ufc.br
2. Evandro Chagas National Institute of Infectious Diseases, Oswaldo Cruz Foundation, Rio de Janeiro, RJ 21040-360, Brazil; andrea.silvestre@ini.fiocruz.br
3. Department of Community Health and Postgraduate Course in Public Health, School of Medicine, Federal University of Ceará, Fortaleza, CE 60430-140, Brazil
* Correspondence: heukelbach@ufc.br

Keywords: Chagas disease; American trypanosomiasis; *Trypanosoma cruzi* infection; neglected tropical disease; public health; epidemiology; prevention and control; surveillance; clinical research; One Health

Despite being described for the first time more than 110 years ago, Chagas disease persists as one of the most neglected tropical diseases. There are limited new treatment options, and diagnosis, surveillance, and control face major bottlenecks. Morbidity and mortality are still high in many settings, both in endemic and non-endemic areas.

This Special Issue of *Tropical Medicine and Infectious Diseases* contains a total of 14 peer-reviewed papers (one editorial, eight original papers, three reviews, one case report, and one opinion paper). The papers span a variety of disciplines and contribute significantly to reduce the gap in scientific knowledge on Chagas disease, towards the Sustainable Development Goals by 2030 [1].

In their editorial, Simone Kropf and Nísia Lima (the current president of the Oswaldo Cruz Foundation in Rio de Janeiro—the first woman in this position) highlight the importance of the recent introduction of the 14th April as the World Chagas Disease Day [2]. On that day in 1909, human infection with *Trypanosoma cruzi* infection was first identified by Carlos Chagas in Brazil. The authors make a strong point for the importance of celebrating this day as a social symbol of science and tropical medicine, focusing on underprivileged and neglected populations in rural hinterlands, being generated not only from European universities, but also by scientists from endemic areas. In this context, the 14th April is also a call for health as a right for all, and for breaking the vicious circle of infectious diseases and poverty. This day may help to give a voice to people at risk, recently organized in an important movement: the International Federation of Associations of People Affected by Chagas Disease (http://findechagas.org/home-en/; accessed on 7 February 2021).

Some papers of this Special Issue focus on health systems and control programs, health care rights, and the burden of Chagas disease for the societies in endemic areas. In most countries, acute disease is of compulsory notification on a national level, but not chronic Chagas disease. Thus, Rocha Siriano et al. [3] highlight the importance of mandatory notification also of chronic Chagas disease to improve the surveillance and follow-up of affected people for comprehensive care. They describe the implementation process of mandatory notification of the disease in the Brazilian state of Goiás. This state lies in the endemic region, with high morbidity and mortality burdens, and has been the pioneer for compulsory notification of chronic Chagas disease since 2013. Since February 2020, chronic disease is of mandatory notification nationwide in Brazil. Premature death related to Chagas disease not only causes suffering for individuals and their families, but also a significant national economic burden, as shown by Olivera et al. [4]. They examined the potential years of work lost, and productivity costs caused by Chagas disease in Colombia, and showed the social significance, making an additional strong point for the strengthening of control programs within the realm of early diagnosis and treatment. Sagenito et al. [5] show that despite being an important public health problem, Chagas disease research is heavily underfunded. Less than 1% of funding and financial support for research on neglected tropical diseases has been allocated to Chagas disease initiatives. This paper shows that the disease is not only being neglected by society and health care workers, but also by policy makers and funding agencies. Another study from Brazil highlights the importance of social, cultural, health system access, and human rights aspects regarding Chagas disease in a highly vulnerable group—Bolivian immigrants to Brazil [6]. While in Brazil healthcare as a human right is guaranteed by the Constitution, including for immigrants, the authors show that in practice, immigrants encounter high barriers for diagnosis and treatment against Chagas disease, such as the regular residency permit, and make a call for the implementation of multidisciplinary teams considering specific social and cultural needs, based on human rights.

Other papers focus on clinical and therapeutic aspects. In their cohort study on children and adolescents from the Brazilian Amazon region, Neves Pinto et al. [7] describe the clinical features of acute and chronic Chagas disease in this population, and the positive effect of the early management of cardiac complications. Their data indicate the effectiveness of treatment for people living in outreach areas. In another paper, Hasslocher-Moreno et al. [8] describe a progression rate of about 7% from the indeterminate to the chronic form of the disease, in a 22-year cohort study, which is lower than usually expected. In an opinion paper, Mendes et al. [9] discuss the importance of the IPEC-FIOCRUZ score—a tool for identifying patients at higher risk—for the prophylaxis against cardioembolic stroke, in patients with Chagas disease. In a retrospective analysis also from Brazil, Rossi Neto et al. [10] suggest that benznidazole may be an effective prophylactic treatment against Chagas disease reactivation in immunosuppressed patients having undergone heart transplantation. Incidence of Chagas disease reactivation in patients receiving benznidazole was 11%, as compared to 46% in patients without prophylaxis. This study reinforces the need for systematic monitoring for Chagas disease reactivation after heart transplantation, and calls for specific randomized double-blinded controlled trials. A case report presents a patient with leishmaniasis and Chagas disease co-infection, and the treatment with meglumine antimoniate which modulated the patient's immune response against both diseases positively [11].

In an entomological survey, Tustin et al. [12] focused on the infection of triatome bugs with *T. cruzi*. They showed that the prevalence of infection in bugs from residences in Peru increased with stage, and that the prevalence in bugs is associated with the number of bites.

In addition, there are three reviews in this Special Issue. First, José Luis Ramirez describes the history of the discovery of the *T. cruzi* genome about 15 years ago, the participation of Latin American researchers, and the implication for Chagas disease research, such as the elaboration of new diagnostic tools [13]. Another review focuses on the reactivation of Chagas disease after heart transplantation [14]. Thirdly, Moll-Bernardes et al. [15] review imaging modalities to detect myocardial fibrosis, inflammation and sympathetic denervation related to Chagas disease—specific factors related to ventricular arrhythmia and sudden death.

This Special Issue provides additional insights into several aspects of Chagas disease, which is still persisting as a public health problem in many Latin American countries. The recently launched new WHO roadmap (Ending the neglect to attain the Sustainable Development Goals: A road map for neglected tropical diseases 2021–2030) [1] defines Chagas disease as one of the diseases in this group targeted for elimination as a public health problem by 2030. This means that 15 countries will have to achieve interruption of transmission through the four main transmission routes (vector, transfusion, transplantation, and congenital transmission), with 75% antiparasitic treatment coverage of the target population. Faced with these new challenges, the coming years will require strong integrated approaches including different aspects, such as evidence-based guidelines, access to healthcare, and human rights [16].

The provided information in this Special Issue will contribute to better understanding several aspects of Chagas disease. The diversity of papers and the new information provided evidence the need for further investment and interdisciplinary work. In fact, Chagas disease is a paradigmatic example for the application of the multidisciplinary One Health approach, to improve its control measures and to reach the elimination goals. The disease encompasses aspects of all four One Health determinant groups related to infection and severe morbidity [17]: firstly, Chagas disease is strongly related to factors involving people and society (including poverty, social inequality, and inadequate living conditions); secondly, animal health plays an important role (such as the presence of wild animals serving as reservoirs, and destruction of natural habitats, increasing the risk of zoonotic transmission); thirdly, governance and health systems are pivotal factors (including vulnerable national and local health systems, inadequate diagnostic capabilities, insufficient surveillance systems, limited priorities of decision makers, and little research funding); and fourthly, the environment, deforestation, and climate change are additional drivers not only for vector transmission, but also for foodborne/oral transmission. Consequently, intensified operational and implementation research efforts are needed to identify the optimal interventions and bottlenecks of control programs, for each specific setting. We are pleased to share the content with the international scientific community, and dedicate this Special Issue to the most underprivileged populations suffering from this and other neglected tropical diseases in Latin America and elsewhere around the globe.

Author Contributions: Writing—original draft preparation, J.H.; writing—review and editing, J.H., A.S.d.S., A.N.R.J.; All authors have read and agreed to the published version of the manuscript.

Funding: This work received no external funding.

Institutional Review Board Statement: Not applicable.

Informed Consent Statement: Not applicable.

Data Availability Statement: Not applicable.

Conflicts of Interest: The authors declare no conflict of interest.

References

1. WHO. *Ending the Neglect to Attain the Sustainable Development Goals: A Road Map for Neglected Tropical Diseases 2021–2030*; World Health Organization: Geneva, Switzerland, 2021.
2. Kropf, P.S.; Lima, T.N. The 14th of April, past and present. *Trop. Med. Infect. Dis.* **2020**, *5*, 100. [CrossRef] [PubMed]
3. da Rocha Siriano, L.; Marchiol, A.; Certo, P.M.; Cubides, J.-C.; Forsyth, C.; de Sousa, A.F. Mandatory notification of chronic chagas disease: Confronting the epidemiological silence in the State of Goiás, Brazil. *Trop. Med. Infect. Dis.* **2020**, *5*, 92. [CrossRef] [PubMed]
4. Olivera, M.J.; Palencia-Sánchez, F.; Riaño-Casallas, M. The cost of lost productivity due to premature chagas disease-related mortality: Lessons from Colombia (2010–2017). *Trop. Med. Infect. Dis.* **2021**, *6*, 17. [CrossRef] [PubMed]
5. Sangenito, L.S.; Branquinha, M.H.; Santos, A.L.S. Funding for chagas disease: A 10-year (2009–2018) survey. *Trop. Med. Infect. Dis.* **2020**, *5*, 88. [CrossRef] [PubMed]
6. Aith, F.M.A.; Forsyth, C.; Shikanai-Yasuda, M.A. Chagas disease and healthcare rights in the bolivian immigrant community of São Paulo, Brazil. *Trop. Med. Infect. Dis.* **2020**, *5*, 62. [CrossRef] [PubMed]
7. Neves Pinto, A.Y.D.; Valente, V.D.C.; Valente, S.A.D.S.; Motta, T.A.R.; Ventura, A.M.R.D.S. Clinical, cardiological and serologic follow-up of chagas disease in children and adolescents from the Amazon Region, Brazil: Longitudinal study. *Trop. Med. Infect. Dis.* **2020**, *5*, 139. [CrossRef] [PubMed]
8. Hasslocher-Moreno, A.M.; Xavier, S.S.; Saraiva, M.R.; Sangenis, C.L.H.; de Holanda, T.M.; Veloso, H.H.; da Costa, R.A.; de Mendes, S.N.S.F.; do Brasil, A.A.P.E.; da Silva, S.G.M.; et al. Progression rate from the indeterminate form to the cardiac form in patients with chronic chagas disease: Twenty-two-year follow-up in a Brazilian urban cohort. *Trop. Med. Infect. Dis.* **2020**, *5*, 76. [CrossRef] [PubMed]

9. Mendes, F.D.S.N.S.; Mediano, M.F.F.; Silva, R.S.; Xavier, S.S.; do Brasil, P.E.A.A.; Saraiva, R.M.; Hasslocher-Moreno, A.M.; de Sousa, A.S. Discussing the score of cardioembolic ischemic stroke in chagas disease. *Trop. Med. Infect. Dis.* **2020**, *5*, 82. [CrossRef] [PubMed]
10. Neto, R.J.M.; Finger, M.A.; dos Santos, C.C. Benznidazole as prophylaxis for chagas disease infection reactivation in heart transplant patients: A case series in Brazil. *Trop. Med. Infect. Dis.* **2020**, *5*, 132. [CrossRef] [PubMed]
11. Rezende-Oliveira, K.; Gómez-Hernández, C.; Silva, M.V.D.; de Oliveira, F.R.; Machado, R.J.; de Teixeira, A.S.L.; Castellano, L.R.C.; Correia, D.; Rodrigues, V. Effects of meglumine antimoniate treatment on cytokine production in a patient with mucosal leishmaniasis and chagas diseases co-infection. *Trop. Med. Infect. Dis.* **2020**, *5*, 69. [CrossRef] [PubMed]
12. Tustin, A.W.; Castillo-Neyra, R.; Tamayo, L.D.; Salazar, R.; Borini-Mayorí, K.; Levy, M.Z. Elucidating the mechanism of trypanosoma cruzi acquisition by triatomine insects: Evidence from a large field survey of triatoma infestans. *Trop. Med. Infect. Dis.* **2020**, *5*, 87. [CrossRef] [PubMed]
13. Ramirez, J.L. *Trypanosoma cruzi* genome 15 years later: What has been accomplished? *Trop. Med. Infect. Dis.* **2020**, *5*, 129. [CrossRef] [PubMed]
14. Moreira, M.d.C.V.; Cunha-Melo, R.J. Chagas disease infection reactivation after heart transplant. *Trop. Med. Infect. Dis.* **2020**, *5*, 106. [CrossRef] [PubMed]
15. Moll-Bernardes, R.J.; Rosado-de-Castro, P.H.; Camargo, G.C.; Mendes, F.S.N.S.; Brito, A.S.X.; Sousa, A.S. New imaging parameters to predict sudden cardiac death in chagas disease. *Trop. Med. Infect. Dis.* **2020**, *5*, 74. [CrossRef] [PubMed]
16. Ramos-Junior, A.N.; Sousa, A.S. The continuous challenge of chagas disease treatment: Bridging evidence-based guidelines, access to healthcare, and human rights. *Rev. Soc. Bras. Med. Trop.* **2017**, *50*, 745–747. [CrossRef] [PubMed]
17. Heukelbach, J. One health & implementation research: Improving health for all. *One Health Implement. Res.* **2020**, *1*, 1–3. [CrossRef]

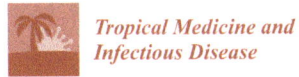

Editorial

The 14th of April, Past and Present

Simone Petraglia Kropf * and Nísia Trindade Lima

Oswaldo Cruz Foundation (Fiocruz), Rio de Janeiro 21040-360, Brazil; nisia.lima@fiocruz.br
* Correspondence: simone.kropf@fiocruz.br

Received: 3 June 2020; Accepted: 11 June 2020; Published: 18 June 2020

In May 2019, the World Health Organization established the "World Chagas Disease Day", to be celebrated on the 14th of April. But why choose this date?

Those who are familiar with the history of Chagas disease know that this was the day that Carlos Ribeiro Justiniano Chagas first identified the *Trypanosoma cruzi* infection in a human being, namely the two-year-old girl Berenice Soares de Moura [1–3]. Ironically, despite going down in history as the first described case of the new trypanosomiasis, discovered in the hinterlands of Brazil in 1909, she would live for many decades without developing any symptoms of the disease, passing away at 72 years of age due to neurological causes unrelated to Chagas disease.

The landmark discovery, which now frames the "World Chagas Disease Day", has a significance that goes beyond chronology. Like any memory rite, it recovers and monumentalizes the past from the horizons and perspectives of the present, as well as the future that one wants to project. What, then, is this significance? Why "celebrate" (in the sense of "remembering together") April 14th?

First, it concerns a celebration of science, by paying homage to a long and successful tradition of research produced in Brazil, that has achieved wide national and international recognition since the beginning [1,3]. It represents clear evidence that Brazilian scientists were, and are, not mere consumers or recipients of theories and ideas coming from European centers, but active subjects (albeit under asymmetric relations) in the production of knowledge [1,3–5]. Tropical medicine, of which Chagas disease would become an emblem, went through a decisive moment of institutionalization in the country at the time, which was a direct result of the establishment of the Oswaldo Cruz Institute (the origin of what is now the Oswaldo Cruz Foundation) [3,5–7]. It is worth mentioning that this happened only a few years after the creation of the first schools and institutes dedicated to this specialty in Europe.

If the past evoked by memory gains meaning in the present, giving global visibility to this landmark of Brazilian science becomes a political act of affirmation to its importance, not only as an activity that advances the frontiers of knowledge, but as a practice intended to provide solutions to concrete social problems, which requires expertise and actions at local, but also global levels.

In this sense, it projects the value of a scientific tradition deeply committed to the health of historically neglected populations onto the world scene. The science that described a new disease in the small town of Lassance would also describe a different country, the 'Brazil of the hinterlands', marked by abandonment and plagued by this and so many other diseases. This was a Brazil quite different from the one that was enjoyed by the elites, who celebrated progress on the French-like avenues in the recently remodeled capital Rio de Janeiro [8]. As Carlos Chagas said since his early work: If Europeans studied tropical diseases because they considered them an obstacle to their colonialist enterprise, studying American trypanosomiasis and other parasitic diseases in Brazil was important because they affected the health of its own populations [9,10]. Understanding and fighting these diseases was, therefore, a central element in a broader project for the construction of a new Brazil [3,8].

This takes us to the second dimension of the significance of the 14th of April: its social meaning, literally embodied in the encounter that took place in 1909. When examining Berenice, who lived in a miserable hut that was infested by triatomine bugs (or 'kissing bugs'), Carlos Chagas did not just find the parasite he was looking for, but also the tangible and human face of poverty. It was the first of many such faces that he would encounter from then on, which revealed to him the structural "social parasitism" gnawing away at the country through its heritage of colonialism and slavery, as the physician Manoel Bomfim argued in his book "Latin America: evils of origin", an important work of Brazilian social thought [11].

Carlos Chagas would not tire of saying that disease and poverty were two sides of the same coin, a problem for which the solution depended on the State's firm action in the implementation of public health policies, aiming to serve Berenice and so many others affected by what he called "diseases of Brazil" [3,5,10,12]. When assuming the leadership of the federal health services ten years later, the scientist from the Oswaldo Cruz Institute would put these ideas into practice by bringing health services and policies to remote corners of Brazil, serving populations that had never seen any sign of public authorities [13]. Therefore, remembering the 14th of April has a political meaning, defending a conception of health as a right of the people and a duty of the State [12].

In the 110 years that have passed since the discovery of Chagas disease, many advances have been made in understanding and coping with this disease, not only in Brazil, but also in other countries [14]. However, despite these advances, the disease still affects an estimated 8 million people worldwide, who, like Berenice, were and are neglected. The biggest challenge, and the main reason for the importance of the 14th of April, is to give visibility to these people, as Carlos Chagas did. But not only that, it is a question of giving them a voice and a leading role, so that they are able to be included as active subjects in the collective undertaking of science and health initiatives aimed at serving them [15].

Experiencing the World Chagas Disease Day amid the COVID-19 pandemic, an emerging disease caused by the coronavirus SARS-CoV-2, gives the date a unique and dramatic tone. May the current health emergency, which mobilizes the world for the imperative need to support science and health, be an occasion to reflect on the structural problems that we have been facing for so many decades as well. May the 14th of April 2020 be an invitation to understand that the path is one: Science in service of health and life, for people with faces and names, like Berenice.

Conflicts of Interest: The authors declare no conflict of interest.

References

1. Kropf, S.K.; Sá, M.R. The discovery of *Trypanosoma cruzi* and Chagas disease (1908–1909): Tropical medicine in Brazil. *História Ciências Saúde-Manguinhos* **2009**, *16*, 13–34. [CrossRef] [PubMed]
2. Kropf, S.P.; Lacerda, A.L. *Carlos Chagas, a Scientist of Brazil*; Editora Fiocruz: Rio de Janeiro, Brazil, 2009.
3. Kropf, S.P. *Doença de Chagas, Doença do Brasil: Ciência, Saúde e Nação (1909–1962)*; Editora Fiocruz: Rio de Janeiro, Brazil, 2009.
4. Kropf, S.P.; Azevedo, N.; Ferreira, L.O. Biomedical Research and public health in Brazil: The case of Chagas disease (1909–1950). *Soc. Hist. Med.* **2003**, *6*, 111–129. [CrossRef]
5. Kropf, S.P. Chagas disease in Brazil: Historical aspects. In *Chagas Disease: Still a Threat to Our World?* Gadelha, F.R., Peloso, E.F., Eds.; Nova Science Publishers: New York, NY, USA, 2013; pp. 1–21.
6. Stepan, N.L. *Beginnings of Brazilian Science: Oswaldo Cruz, Medical Research and Policy, 1890–1920*; Science History Publications, Neale Watson Academic Publ. Inc.: New York, NY, USA, 1976.
7. Kropf, S.K. Tropical Medicine in Brazil. *Wellcome Hist.* **2011**, *47*, 18–19.
8. Lima, N.T. *Um Sertão Chamado Brasil: Intelectuais e Representação Geográfica da Identidade Nacional*; Revan/IUPERJ: Rio de Janeiro, Brazil, 1999.
9. Chagas, C. *Cadeira de Medicina Tropical*; Aula inaugural do Prof. Carlos Chagas, no Pavilhão Miguel Couto, a 14 de setembro de 1926; Typografia do IOC: Rio de Janeiro, Brazil, 1926.
10. Kropf, S.P. Carlos Chagas e as doenças do Brasil. In *Médicos Intérpretes do Brasil*; Hochman, G., Lima, N.T., Eds.; Hucitec: São Paulo, Brazil, 2015; pp. 194–222.
11. Bomfim, M. *A América Latina: Males de Origem, [online]*; Centro Edelstein de Pesquisas Sociais: Rio de Janeiro, Brazil, 2008; [first edition in 1905].

12. Kropf, S.P. Carlos Chagas: Science, health and national debate in Brazil. *Lancet (Br. Ed.)* **2011**, *377*, 1740–1741. [CrossRef]
13. Hochman, G. *The Sanitation of Brazil. Nation, State and Public Health*; University of Illinois Press: Urbana-Champaign, Champaign, IL, USA, 2016.
14. Carvalheiro, J.R.; Azevedo, N.; Araújo-Jorge, T.C.; Lannes-Vieira, J.; Soeiro, M.N.; Klein, L. (Eds.) *Clássicos em Doença de Chagas: História e Perspectivas no Centenário da Descoberta*; Editora Fiocruz: Rio de Janeiro, Brazil, 2009.
15. Coura, J.R.; Viñas, P.A. Chagas Disease: A New Worldwide Challenge. *Nature* **2010**, *465*, S6–S7. [CrossRef] [PubMed]

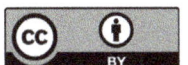

© 2020 by the authors. Licensee MDPI, Basel, Switzerland. This article is an open access article distributed under the terms and conditions of the Creative Commons Attribution (CC BY) license (http://creativecommons.org/licenses/by/4.0/).

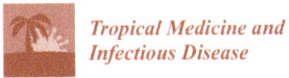

Tropical Medicine and Infectious Disease

Article

The Cost of Lost Productivity Due to Premature Chagas Disease-Related Mortality: Lessons from Colombia (2010–2017)

Mario J. Olivera [1,2,*], Francisco Palencia-Sánchez [3] and Martha Riaño-Casallas [4]

1. Grupo de Parasitología, Instituto Nacional de Salud, Bogotá 111321, D.C., Colombia
2. Programme in Health Economics, Pontificia Universidad Javeriana, Bogotá 110231, D.C., Colombia
3. Facultad de Medicina, Departamento de Medicina Preventiva y Social, Pontificia Universidad Javeriana, Bogotá 110231, D.C., Colombia; fpalencia@javeriana.edu.co
4. Facultad de Ciencias Económicas, Universidad Nacional de Colombia, Bogotá 111321, D.C., Colombia; mirianoc@unal.edu.co
* Correspondence: molivera@ins.gov.co; Tel.: +57-1-220-7700

Abstract: Background: Economic burden due to premature mortality has a negative impact not only in health systems but also in wider society. The aim of this study was to estimate the potential years of work lost (PYWL) and the productivity costs of premature mortality due to Chagas disease in Colombia from 2010 to 2017. Methods: National data on mortality (underlying cause of death) were obtained from the National Administrative Department of Statistics in Colombia between 2010 and 2017, in which Chagas disease was mentioned on the death certificate as an underlying or associated cause of death. Chagas disease as a cause of death corresponded to category B57 (Chagas disease) including all subcategories (B57.0 to B57.5), according to the Tenth Revision of the International Statistical Classification of Diseases and Related Health Problems (ICD-10). The electronic database contains the number of deaths from all causes by sex and 5-year age group. Economic data, including wages, unemployment rates, labor force participation rates and gross domestic product, were derived from the Bank of the Republic of Colombia. The human capital approach was applied to estimate both the PYWL and present value of lifetime income lost due to premature deaths. A discount rate of 3% was applied and results are presented in 2017 US dollars (USD). Results: There were 1261 deaths in the study, of which, 60% occurred in males. Premature deaths from Chagas resulted in 48,621 PYWL and a cost of USD 29 million in the present value of lifetime income forgone. Conclusion: The productivity costs of premature mortality due to Chagas disease are significant. These results provide an economic measure of the Chagas burden which can help policy makers allocate resources to continue with early detection programs.

Keywords: Chagas disease; cost of illness; premature; efficiency; organizational; life expectancy

Citation: Olivera, M.J.; Palencia-Sánchez, F.; Riaño-Casallas, M. The Cost of Lost Productivity Due to Premature Chagas Disease-Related Mortality: Lessons from Colombia (2010–2017). *Trop. Med. Infect. Dis.* 2021, 6, 17. https://doi.org/10.3390/tropicalmed6010017

Received: 13 April 2020
Accepted: 30 June 2020
Published: 27 January 2021

Publisher's Note: MDPI stays neutral with regard to jurisdictional claims in published maps and institutional affiliations.

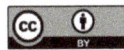

Copyright: © 2021 by the authors. Licensee MDPI, Basel, Switzerland. This article is an open access article distributed under the terms and conditions of the Creative Commons Attribution (CC BY) license (https://creativecommons.org/licenses/by/4.0/).

1. Introduction

Chagas disease remains a serious public health problem worldwide, having serious economic and social repercussions [1]. The infection is endemic in South America and emergent in Europe and the United States [2]. This parasitic disease affects 6–7 million people worldwide, causing more than 7000 deaths each year [3]. The cost of Chagas disease was USD 13.1 million in 2017 [4].

Chagas disease generates a significant health burden for individuals and a large economic burden in low- and middle-income countries in the Americas and in some high-income countries over recent decades [4]. Among the working-age population, the economic cost of illness-related productivity losses as a result of lower productivity at work, lost workdays, and mortality can far exceed the Chagas disease-related medical costs [5].

It is important to quantify the value of the labor productivity loss due to premature mortality in measuring the economic burden of disease. Specially, this metric should be quantified for communicable diseases in that affect low- and middle-income countries. To quantify the cost of economic losses owing to premature death in the working-age population, this value is used as the indicator of years of potential productive life lost [6,7]. In this case, we focused on economic cost. Chagas disease has been associated with excess mortality [8]. The most frequently used measures of economic loss due to premature death are years of potential life lost (YPLL) and potential years of work lost (PYWL) [6,9–11].

Chagas disease is a clear threat not only to human health but also the level of family income and economic growth in a country, particularly in rural areas [4]. It is estimated that 752,000 working years per year are lost due to premature deaths caused by diseases in the seven countries of South America, which corresponds to USD 1208.5 million/year [5].

Despite the high prevalence of Chagas disease estimated in Colombia 2.0% (95% CI: 1.0–4.0) [12], few studies have estimated the productivity losses associated with premature deaths from this infection in the country [4]. Therefore, this study aimed to estimate the PYWL associated with premature deaths caused by Chagas disease during the period from 2010 to 2017 in Colombia.

2. Materials and Methods

This study was developed based on the human capital approach to estimate the costs of productivity derived from premature mortality due to Chagas disease in Colombia. Premature mortality was defined as death from Chagas disease before the age of 62 (for men) or 57 (for women), years old. The human capital approach equates the productivity lost to an individual's wage rate and assumes that an individual produces a stream of output over a working lifetime cut short by premature death. All expenses were reported as Colombian pesos (COP) and were converted to US dollars (1 USD (US$) = 2984 COP) from 2017 [13].

2.1. Data Source

Numbers of deaths in 2010–2017 by 5-year age group and sex between the ages of 15 and 62 were obtained from the mortality database of the National Administrative Department of Statistics (DANE) using the Tenth Revision of the International Statistical Classification of Diseases and Related Health Problems (ICD-10) code B57, including all subcategories (B57.0 to B57.5) [14]. The database contains number of deaths of all causes by sex and 5-year age. Economic data, including wages, unemployment rates, labor force participation rates and gross domestic product (GDP), were derived from Bank of the Republic of Colombia.

2.2. Estimation Methods

The number of deaths that could be attributed to Chagas from 2010 to 2017 by sex was extracted, and from these, PYWL for men and women were determined across the productive age groups (between 18 and 62 years old, retire at 62 (for men) or 57 (for women)—the official pensionable age in Colombia in 2017 [15]). Premature mortality costs involved multiplying, for each death, PYWL by age- and gender-stratified gross wages from age of death until to the official pensionable age. Estimates were the adjusted probability of being in work. Wage growth was calculated at 2.5% per annum, and a discount rate of 3% annually was applied. The scenario that assessed the 2017 minimum annual salary (USD 3301 per year) was modeled. In Colombia on average the growth of the real wage was 2%. Statistical analysis was performed using Stata version 14.0 (Stata Corporation LP, College Station, TX, USA). All variables included in the study were described using the appropriate univariate statistics.

2.3. Sensitivity Analyses

One-way sensitivity analysis was conducted to assess the effects of varying the parameters: the wage growth rate varied from 1.5% to 3.5% to account for uncertainty over future growth in the Colombian economy, and the minimum annual salary between USD 2715 and USD 4000. In addition, the effect of extending the retirement age was explored.

3. Results

From 2010 to 2017, 1446 deaths of Chagas disease were recorded. Of these, 185 deaths occurred in people under 18 years of age were excluded. In total, 1261 deaths were analyzed in the study, of which 60% corresponded to males. The mean age at death was 21 years. Table 1 presents the number of deaths of all ages for males and females. PYWL was lower in women than men (18,384 vs. 30,237), overall PYWL was 48,621. It noticed that the deaths each year of the analysis period.

Table 1. The number of deaths and estimated Potential Years of Work Lost (PYWL) by sex from 2010 to 2017.

Year	2010	2011	2012	2013	2014	2015	2016	2017	Total
				Number of Deaths					
Males	102	87	101	110	113	93	132	128	866
Females	58	51	59	71	79	85	92	85	580
Total	160	138	160	181	192	178	224	213	1446
				Deaths at Working Age					
Males	84	69	88	95	93	83	117	112	741
Females	52	45	51	64	72	76	84	76	520
Total	136	114	139	159	165	159	201	188	1261
				PYWL					
Males	3441	2822	3594	3900	3777	3348	4772	4583	30,237
Females	1854	1593	1824	2263	2521	2682	2968	2679	18,384
Total	5295	4415	5418	6163	6298	6030	7740	7262	48,621

Table 2 demonstrates the average premature mortality per PYWL by sex from 2010 to 2017. The cost per PYWL for both sexes combined was USD 29,683,913 in the study period, and it was USD 17.3 million for males and USD 12.3 million for females from 2010 to 2017. In the case of women, they tended to have lower wages and a shorter working life.

Table 2. Premature mortality cost by sex per death and per Potential Years of Work Lost (PYWL) (USD 2017).

	Total Premature Mortality Cost	% of the Total	Premature Mortality Cost per Death	Premature Mortality Cost per PYWL
Males	17,301,237	58	23,348	572
Females	12,382,676	42	23,813	674
Total	29,683,913	100	23,540	611

The total cost of lost productivity due to premature mortality was 39.7% higher in males than females, although the cost per PYWL was higher in females.

Table 3 shows the cost of premature mortality sex in each year of the period.

Table 3. Premature mortality cost per sex 2010–2017 (USD 2017).

Year	2010	2011	2012	2013	2014	2015	2016	2017
Males	1,862,873	1,541,799	2,008,175	2,198,782	2,206,153	1,986,068	2,793,321	2,704,067
Females	1,174,136	1,023,484	1,183,187	1,509,232	1,736,916	1,846,584	2,040,400	1,868,737
Total	3,037,009	2,565,283	3,191,362	3,708,014	3,943,069	3,832,652	4,833,722	4,572,803

We classified the people included according to age; people who died between the ages of 18 and 25 years were categorized as young and people above 25 years old classified as adults. Therefore, Table 4 shows the impact of the cost is bigger.

Table 4. Premature mortality cost per group age 2010–2017 (USD 2017).

Age Group/Year	2010	2011	2012	2013	2014	2015	2016	2017
Adults	22,597	68,203	46,165	47,106	96,491	72,932	170,012	98,320
Young	3,014,412	2,497,081	3,145,197	3,660,908	3,846,578	3,759,719	4,663,710	4,474,483

Figure 1 shows a boxplot of cost of premature mortality by sex, for which the variation was higher for men per death than for women. This is because men die younger than women and they have a longer pensionable age. In the graph, the circles are outlier values of the cost of PYWL.

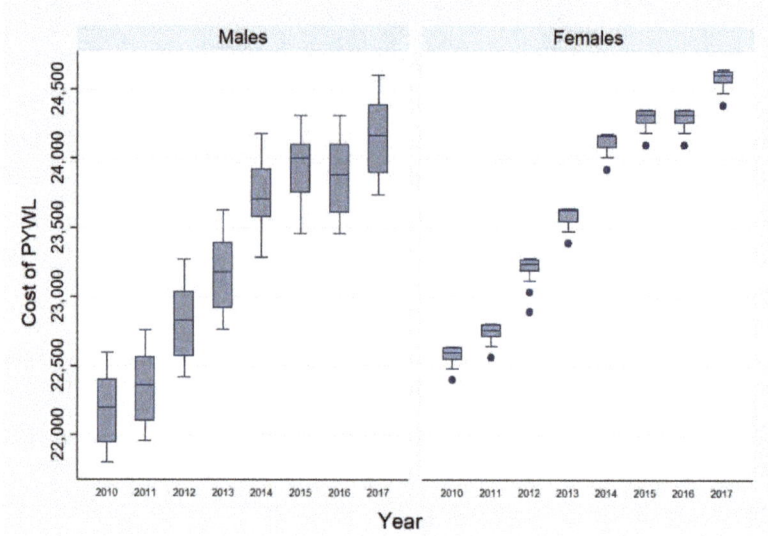

Figure 1. Cost of productivity lost due to premature mortality by sex (USD 2017).

Figure 2 depicts the PYWL per occupational group; construction workers, farm workers and unskilled workers were the groups with the most years lost. In the graph, the circles are outlier values of the cost of PYWL in farm workers.

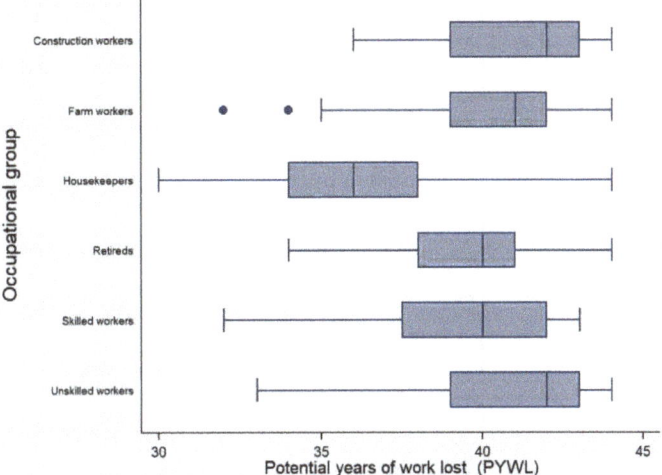

Figure 2. Potential Years of Work Lost (PYWL) by occupation.

4. Discussion

The main finding of this study was the estimation of the monetary value of the accumulated labor productivity losses during the 2010–2017 period due to deaths caused by Chagas disease in Colombia. This cost amounted to USD 29 million. Despite the magnitude of the estimated cost, the trend observed throughout the period was that of further increasing costs. However, it should be clarified that this increase in the number of deaths could be due to the strengthening of surveillance systems that allow for a better counting of deaths and to the strengthening of the health system.

In recent years, Colombia has had great social, demographic, environmental and technological transformations in a sustained manner, and despite the innumerable situations of social injustice, the living conditions of the populations have improved significantly [16,17]. However, diseases associated with contexts of social vulnerability and neglect, such as Chagas disease, still affect a considerable part of the population for example workers such as unskilled workers, farm worker and construction workers [12].

It is also worrying that the percentage of deaths from preventable Chagas disease continues to be high in the younger population. This is probably associated with barriers to timely diagnosis that persist in the country and the difficulties associated with treatment [1,18,19]. This implies support for the early detection programs [20,21].

Interestingly, 60% of the estimated losses in labor productivity can be attributed to men. This can be explained by the higher risk of death in this group and, on the other hand, by the fact that employment rates and wages were higher for men than for women. It could also be related to the difference between men and women. These results are concordantwith previous studies that have consistently reported that men have a higher risk of death than women [22,23].

Previous studies have tried to estimate the social impact of premature deaths on workers suffering from Chagas disease, but over a short time period [4]. On the other hand, some research has delved into the loss of health-related quality of life caused by the consequences of the disease [24,25]. The strengthening and implementation of public policies aimed at eliminating barriers to early diagnosis and treatment of Chagas disease can impact on the reduction of mortality [26].

It is important to note that the theoretical approach used in the present study is ttheory of human capital [27]. The main alternative approach is the so-called friction-cost method [28]. Although the methodological discussion on the strengths and weaknesses of both approaches has been intense, there is still no agreement on which is best [27]. In this study, the human capital approach was chosen due to its greater anchorage with economic theory and it is the most widely used method in the scientific literature on disease cost studies.

The main limitations include, firstly, the real wages of people killed by Chagas disease (estimated from the average wage in Colombia) were not considered. Second, there was also no information on whether the deceased worked or not (the average employment rates adjusted for age and sex). Third, the mortality database might have been vastly underreported in official statistics.

5. Conclusions

Reducing premature and preventable deaths from Chagas disease is a key health goal in the ten-year plan for Colombian public health. The size of the economic impact and the burden on society due to premature deaths from Chagas disease reinforces the need to continue investing in early detection programs, as well as initiatives that promote prosperity and well-being for all.

Author Contributions: All authors contributed equally to the design of the study, data collection, data analysis, data interpretation, and manuscript writing, and all authors have read and agreed to the published version of the manuscript. Conceptualization, M.J.O., F.P.-S. and M.R.-C.; methodology, M.J.O., F.P.-S. and M.R.-C., software, M.J.O., F.P.-S. and M.R.-C.; validation, M.J.O., F.P.-S. and M.R.-C.; formal analysis, M.J.O., F.P.-S. and M.R.-C. investigation, M.J.O., F.P.-S. and M.R.-C.; resources, M.J.O., F.P.-S. and M.R.-C.; data curation, M.J.O., F.P.-S. and M.R.-C.; writing—original draft preparation, M.J.O., F.P.-S. and M.R.-C.; writing—review and editing, M.J.O., F.P.-S. and M.R.-C.; visualization, M.J.O., F.P.-S. and M.R.-C.; supervision, M.J.O., F.P.-S. and M.R.-C.; project administration, M.J.O., F.P.-S. and M.R.-C.

Funding: This research received no external funding.

Conflicts of Interest: The authors declare that there is no conflict of interest.

References

1. Olivera, M.J.; Porras, J.; Toquica, C.; Rodríguez, J. Barriers to diagnosis dccess for Chagas disease in Colombia. *J. Parasitol. Res.* **2018**, *2018*, 4940796. [CrossRef] [PubMed]
2. Pinto Dias, J.C. Human Chagas disease and migration in the context of globalization: Some particular aspects. *J. Trop. Med.* **2013**, *2013*, 789758. [CrossRef]
3. World Health Organization. Chagas disease in Latin America: An epidemiological update based on 2010 estimates. *Wkly. Epidemiol. Rec.* **2015**, *90*, 33–44.
4. Olivera, M.J.; Buitrago, G. Economic costs of Chagas disease in Colombia in 2017: A social perspective. *Int. J. Infect. Dis.* **2020**, *91*, 196–201. [CrossRef] [PubMed]
5. World Health Organization. First WHO Report on Neglected Tropical Diseases: Working to Overcome the Global Impact of Neglected Tropical Diseases. France, 2010. Available online: https://www.who.int/neglected_diseases/2010report/en/ (accessed on 6 March 2020).
6. Gardner, J.W.; Sanborn, J.S. Years of potential life lost (YPLL)-What does it measure? *Epidemiology* **1990**, *1*, 322–329. [CrossRef]
7. Darbà, J.; Marsà, A. The cost of lost productivity due to premature lung cancer-related mortality: Results from Spain over a 10-year period. *BMC Cancer* **2019**, *19*, 992. [CrossRef]
8. Cucunubá, Z.M.; Okuwoga, O.; Basáñez, M.G.; Nouvellet, P. Increased mortality attributed to Chagas disease: A systematic review and meta-analysis. *Parasites Vectors* **2016**, *9*, 42. [CrossRef]
9. Wise, R.P.; Livengood, J.R.; Berkelman, R.L.; Goodman, R.A. Methodological alternatives for measuring premature mortality. *Am. J. Prev. Med.* **1988**, *4*, 268–273. [CrossRef]
10. Romeder, J.M.; McWhinnie, J.R. Potential years of life lost between ages 1 and 70: An indicator of premature mortality for health planning. *Int. J. Epidemiol.* **1977**, *6*, 143–151. [CrossRef]
11. Zhong, Y.; Li, D. Potential years of life lost and work tenure lost when silicosis is compared with other pneumoconioses. *Scand. J. Work Environ. Health* **1995**, *21*, 91–94.
12. Olivera, M.J.; Fory, J.A.; Porras, J.F.; Buitrago, G. Prevalence of Chagas disease in Colombia: A systematic review and meta-analysis. *PLoS ONE* **2019**, *14*, e0210156. [CrossRef] [PubMed]
13. Banco de la República Colombia. Tasa Representativa del Mercado (TRM-Peso por dólar). Available online: https://www.banrep.gov.co/es/estadisticas/trm (accessed on 24 February 2020).

14. Departamento Administrativo Nacional de Estadística. Mortalidad en Colombia, 2017. Available online: https://www.dane.gov.co/index.php/estadisticas-por-tema/demografia-y-poblacion/nacimientos-y-defunciones (accessed on 6 March 2020).
15. Congreso de Colombia. Ley 100 de 1993. Por la Cual se Crea el Sistema de Seguridad Social Integral y se Dictan Otras Disposiciones. Available online: http://www.secretariasenado.gov.co/senado/basedoc/ley_0100_1993.html (accessed on 6 March 2020).
16. Augustovski, F.; Alcaraz, A.; Caporale, J.; García Martí, S.; Pichon Riviere, A. Institutionalizing health technology assessment for priority setting and health policy in Latin America: From regional endeavors to national experiences. *Expert Rev. Pharmacoecon. Outcomes Res.* **2015**, *15*, 9–12. [CrossRef] [PubMed]
17. Departamento Administrativo Nacional de Estadística. Encuesta Nacional de Calidad de vida 2018. 2019. Available online: https://www.dane.gov.co/index.php/estadisticas-por-tema/pobreza-y-condiciones-de-vida/calidad-de-vida-ecv (accessed on 6 March 2020).
18. Olivera, M.J.; Cucunuba, Z.M.; Alvarez, C.A.; Nicholls, R.S. Safety profile of nifurtimox and treatment interruption for chronic Chagas disease in Colombian adults. *Am. J. Trop. Med. Hyg.* **2015**, *93*, 1224–1230. [CrossRef] [PubMed]
19. Olivera, M.J.; Cucunuba, Z.M.; Valencia-Hernandez, C.A.; Herazo, R.; Agreda-Rudenko, D.; Florez, C.; Duque, S.; Nicholls, R.S. Risk factors for treatment interruption and severe adverse effects to benznidazole in adult patients with Chagas disease. *PLoS ONE* **2017**, *12*, e0185033. [CrossRef] [PubMed]
20. Olivera, M.J.; Fory, J.A.; Olivera, A.J. Quality assessment of clinical practice guidelinesfor Chagas disease. *Rev. Soc. Bras. Med. Trop.* **2015**, *48*, 343–346. [CrossRef] [PubMed]
21. Olivera, M.J.; Fory, J.A.; Olivera, A.J. Therapeutic drug monitoring of benznidazole and nifurtimox: A systematic review and quality assessment of published clinical practice guidelines. *Rev. Soc. Bras. Med. Trop.* **2017**, *50*, 748–755. [CrossRef]
22. Basquiera, A.L.; Sembaj, A.; Aguerri, A.M.; Omelianiuk, M.; Guzmán, S.; Moreno Barral, J.; Caeiro, T.F.; Madoery, R.J.; Salomone, O.A. Risk progression to chronic Chagas cardiomyopathy: Influence of male sex and of parasitaemia detected by polymerase chain reaction. *Heart* **2003**, *89*, 1186–1190. [CrossRef]
23. Sabino, E.C.; Ribeiro, A.L.; Salemi, V.M.C.; Di Lorenzo Oliveira, C.; Antunes, A.P.; Menezes, M.M.; Lanni, B.M.; Nastari, L.; Fernandes, F.; Patavino, G.M.; et al. Ten-year incidence of Chagas cardiomyopathy among asymptomatic trypanosoma cruzi-seropositive former blood donors. *Circulation* **2013**, *127*, 1105–1115. [CrossRef]
24. Pelegrino, V.M.; Dantas, R.A.S.; Ciol, M.A.; Clark, A.M.; Rossi, L.A.; Simoes, M.V. Health-related quality of life in Brazilian outpatients with Chagas and non-Chagas cardiomyopathy. *Heart Lung* **2011**, *40*, e25–e31. [CrossRef]
25. Oliveira, B.G.; Abreu, M.N.S.; Abreu, C.D.G.; da Costa Rocha, M.O.; Ribeiro, A.L. Health-related quality of life in patients with Chagas disease. *Rev. Soc. Bras. Med. Trop.* **2011**, *44*, 150–156. [CrossRef]
26. Olivera, M.J.; Chaverra, K.A. New diagnostic algorithm for Chagas disease: Impact on access to diagnosis and out-of-pocket expenditures in Colombia. *Iran. J. Public Health* **2019**, *48*, 1379–1381. [CrossRef] [PubMed]
27. Drummond, M.; Sculpher, M.; Claxton, K.; Stoddart, G.; Torrance, G. *Methods for the Economic Evaluation of Health Care Programmes*, 4th ed.; Oxford University Press: Oxford, UK, 2015.
28. Pike, J.; Grosse, S.D. Friction cost estimates of productivity costs in cost-of-illness studies in comparison with human capital estimates: A review. *Appl. Health Econ. Health Policy* **2018**, *16*, 765–778. [CrossRef] [PubMed]

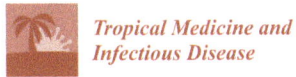

Article

Mandatory Notification of Chronic Chagas Disease: Confronting the Epidemiological Silence in the State of Goiás, Brazil

Liliane da Rocha Siriano [1,*], Andrea Marchiol [2], Marina Pereira Certo [2,*], Juan-Carlos Cubides [3], Colin Forsyth [2] and Fabrício Augusto de Sousa [1]

[1] State Coordination of Zoonoses, Epidemiological Surveillance Management (GVE), Health Surveillance Superintendence (SUVISA), Goiás State Health Secretary (SES), Goiânia 74093-250, Brazil; zoonoses.go.gov@gmail.com
[2] Access Project and Operational Research Platform for Chagas, Drugs for Neglected Diseases initiative (DNDi), Rio de Janeiro 20010-903, Brazil; amarchiol@dndi.org (A.M.); cforsyth@dndi.org (C.F.)
[3] Brazilian Medical Unit-BRAMU, Doctors without Borders (MSF), Rio de Janeiro 20040-006, Brazil; juan.cubides@rio.msf.org
* Correspondence: liliane.siriano@yahoo.com.br (L.d.R.S.); mcerto@dndi.org (M.P.C.)

Received: 9 April 2020; Accepted: 1 June 2020; Published: 5 June 2020

Abstract: Objectives: This paper presents the results of the design and implementation process for the policy of compulsory notification of chronic Chagas disease in the Brazilian state of Goiás (Resolution No. 004/2013-GAB/SES-GO). Methods: The narrative was based on information provided by key actors that were part of the different stages of the process, built on contextual axes based on participants' reflections about the establishment of the most accurate and coherent notification mechanisms. Results: The notification policy addressed the absence of historical data from patients in the state Chagas program, an increase in cases identified through serology, and weaknesses in vector control. Two key challenges involved human resources capacity and dissemination to public agencies and health care workers. Effective training and communication processes were key ingredients for successful implementation. Conclusions: The lack of public health measures aimed at the epidemiological surveillance of chronic Chagas cases constitutes a significant barrier for patients to access appropriate diagnosis, management and follow-up, and hampers the planning of necessary activities within health systems. The implementation of the notification policy in Goiás allows authorities to determine the real magnitude of Chagas disease in the population, so that an appropriate public health response can be mounted to meet the needs of affected people, thereby ending the epidemiological silence of Chagas disease.

Keywords: Chagas disease; disease notification; public policy; neglected topical diseases; healthcare access

1. Introduction

Chagas disease is classified by the World Health Organization (WHO) as part of the Neglected Tropical Diseases (NTDs) group [1]. NTDs are characterized not only by their substantial social impact in various settings throughout the world but also by gaps in epidemiological surveillance and a lack of effective diagnostic and therapeutic tools to bolster control initiatives [2]. There are relatively scarce epidemiological data available for these often-hidden diseases, making it difficult to accurately assess their burden, and impairing the ability of governments to respond with appropriate public policies.

The International Statistical Classification of Diseases and Related Health Problems (ICD) systematizes data for Chagas disease and other conditions. This classification is based on a notification system, defined as the communication to public health authorities of the existence of a disease in humans. The purpose of this communication is to understand the magnitude and epidemiological characteristics, as well as establish control measures to prevent the spread of diseases. This information also enables the planning, execution, and evaluation of publicly controlled policies. The case of Chagas disease is especially complex due to its particular biological context (with a typically unrecognizable acute phase and long asymptomatic period) and social dimensions (primarily affecting marginalized populations including migrants and the rural poor). These conditions, along with severe gaps in diagnostic coverage, make it difficult to monitor current surveillance systems.

Reporting of the acute form of Chagas disease is mandatory in Brazil, as it is for any other disease with an acute presentation with significant morbidity and mortality [3]. However, in its chronic form, notification of Chagas disease is not mandatory in most endemic countries. This could represent a barrier in surveillance systems in terms of detection, monitoring, and health interventions considering early diagnosis and treatment [4]. The occurrence of a greater socioeconomic and public health impact of the disease is documented in its chronic phase [5]. Moreover, the vast majority of cases are not detected during the acute phase. While the regional incidence in the Americas has declined to around 30,000 annually [6], there are around six million people with chronic infection, the vast majority undiagnosed. The lack of policies supporting notification of chronic cases generates a series of limitations and loss of information for surveillance systems in endemic countries, leading to an epidemiological silence or ignorance of the epidemiological situation of the disease, hampering public policy responses for the benefit of affected populations.

Incomplete and non-systematized information leads to the impossibility of evaluating potential risk scenarios, with regional implications. There are several barriers in this regard, ranging from the problems of endemic regions to the newly emerging urban and cross-border contexts, with a high flow of migrant populations. Other difficulties are found in the definition of specific targets for control programs under national and international commitments and in the exchange of information for analysis and response to new and emerging epidemiological contexts (such as oral transmission and rural-urban and transnational migration). Currently, epidemiological data provided by countries originate mainly from blood blanks, which since the 1980s have complied with specific legislation for universal screening. Other sources of information include community testing activities, serological surveys, certification initiatives for the control of vector transmission of infection and isolated interventions of academic interest [6]. However, these sources provide a largely fragmented picture of the epidemiological burden of the disease.

Brazil has made substantial progress in terms of controlling vector transmission in the last 25 years, reaching the interruption of intra-household vector transmission by *Triatoma infestans* in 2006 [7], although the state of Goiás received this certification in March 2000 [8]. Despite significant efforts to achieve these objectives, Chagas disease remains a significant public health problem in Goiás. Moraes et al. found that 14.8% of all deaths reported in the country due to Chagas disease between 2006 and 2011 were in Goiás, with the state's mortality rate being five times higher in comparison to the rest of the Brazilian territory [9]. There was another study on the detection of communicable diseases in pregnant women in the state of Goiás. It revealed that between 2003 and 2009, 1768 seropositive people were seropositive for *Trypanosoma cruzi* infection, representing 0.5% seroprevalence [10].

Since 2013, Goiás has implemented a mandatory public notification policy at the state level for cases of chronic Chagas disease, which has served as a key contributor in the epidemiological surveillance system, improving awareness of Chagas disease. This policy undoubtedly contributed to Brazil's decision in early 2020 to make Chagas disease reportable at the national level and provides an example that can be replicated in other areas with a similar epidemiological profile. The objective of this paper is to present the results of the design and implementation process for the policy of compulsory notification of chronic Chagas disease in the Brazilian state of Goiás.

2. Methods and Materials

A questionnaire was designed containing a total of 30 questions to obtain relevant information to document the process of creating and implementing a notification policy in Goiás for chronic Chagas cases. The questions were classified into main information groups based on the stages of the public policy formulation cycle model [11].

Four main axes were chosen for data collection: the initial context, to establish how the need/problem was identified; policy design and approval, aiming to identify key actors and actions in the process; implementation, describing resources and capabilities; and evaluation of the current situation in the progress of the policy. Figure 1 illustrates the elements analyzed in each information axis. As depicted in Figure 1, the formulation of public policies is a dynamic, cyclical process.

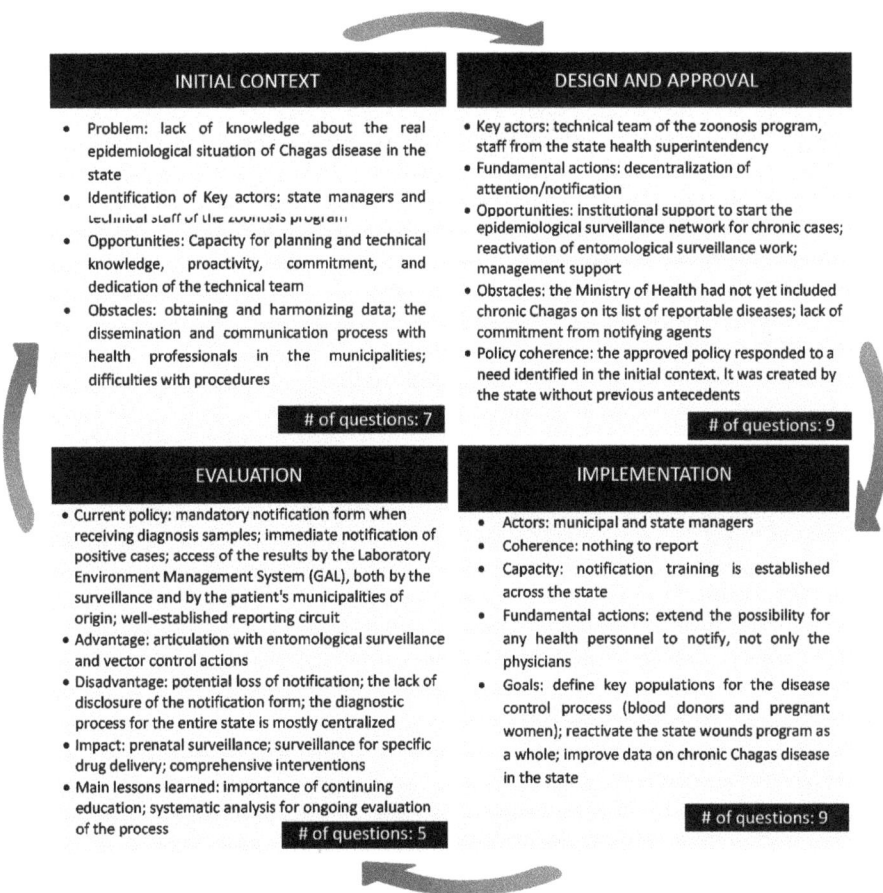

Figure 1. Main information axes for interviews on notification of chronic Chagas disease in Goiás.

A total of seven key employees agreed to participate in the collection of strategic information through the self-administered questionnaire, which was administered during November and December of 2018. Participants were involved in the various operational and management activities of the design and implementation processes of the chronic Chagas case notification policy in Goiás. They had different professional profiles, including two in Biomedicine, one in Biology, one in Nursing, one in

Pharmacy and two from Veterinary Medicine. Most of the questions were open-ended to facilitate the inclusion of details considered pertinent/relevant by the participant.

3. Results

3.1. Initial Context

Six female and one male respondent answered the questionnaire. Respondents spent a time range of 2–8 years in their positions, which were technical (n = 3), managerial (n = 3), or administrative (n = 1). Most interviewees affirmed the notification improved Chagas disease patient access to healthcare completely (n = 5) or at least partially (n = 1); one participant did not answer. Six out of seven felt that improved data and surveillance were necessary to give visibility to the disease. When asked if the notification resolution responded to the needs it was created to address, three completely agreed, three partially agreed, and one did not respond. However, six of seven also affirmed the policy had only been partly implemented as intended.

According to the interviews, the initiative to create the policy for Chronic Chagas Compulsory Notification was consolidated in 2012, motivated mainly by the absence of historical data from patients in the Chagas state program, the increase in cases identified through serology, and the weakening of vector control programs. It was necessary to give visibility to people affected by the disease to define mechanisms for medical care and monitoring and to establish a specialized care network that adequately responded to patients' needs. This entailed having accurate, up-to-date data available. Along with the compulsory notification of chronic patients, a set of actions was proposed to strengthen the state Chagas program.

At the time, the expectation of notification by the municipalities in Goiás was as hopeful as it was challenging. There was a weakened, overloaded notification system for compulsory diseases, characterized by few human resources and high turnover. However, the intention of the specialized team that managed the initiative was to face the need for official data, as well as to raise awareness among municipal teams. This was despite assuming that it would probably be a gradual and slow process and that there was limited recognition of the importance of reporting chronic cases by state and local authorities and managers within the health system. The work carried out to launch the policy creation initiative at the state level took approximately one year, between April 2012 and March 2013.

3.2. Design and Approval

To implement the compulsory notification of chronic Chagas cases, it became necessary to justify the relevance of the information and the impact it would have on epidemiological surveillance at the state level.

The technicians of the area, through internal discussions and with partners from similar areas, were in charge of identifying specific needs through a critical review of the conditions of the state Chagas program. Simultaneously, the team presented potential action items and justifications both to the management of the area and to the superintendence of health surveillance, including the formation of a state care network for patients with Chagas disease, the need to resume work in entomological surveillance in areas in ecosystems with a probability of vector transmission resurgence, and the importance of data to estimate the number of prescriptions and address the inadequate release of medications.

This information gathering instigated a process of discussion and awareness about the need to compulsorily notify cases of chronic Chagas disease, which reached the level of a joint state and municipal health committee. The initiative was also disseminated among the health secretaries of the State of Goiás for their subsequent approval. The process ended with the drafting of the resolution for publication in April 2013.

When assessing whether the public policy resolution would be in accordance with the identified needs, the participants affirmed that it enabled the development of prevention and care actions in relation to the disease as planned, even though there were some initial difficulties in rolling out the new policy. Spreading knowledge of a new policy takes time and requires the adaptation of the professionals involved. Ideally, it would be gradually incorporated into service routines. As part of the dissemination process, the Coordinator of Zoonoses distributed technical note No. 05/2013 to the regional health departments of the state and, consequently, to the municipalities, with guidance on Chagas disease in Goiás, clinical and laboratory diagnosis, control, treatment and compulsory notification in accordance with the approved resolution.

The initiative to create a public notification policy involved several actors at different levels, as described in Figure 2.

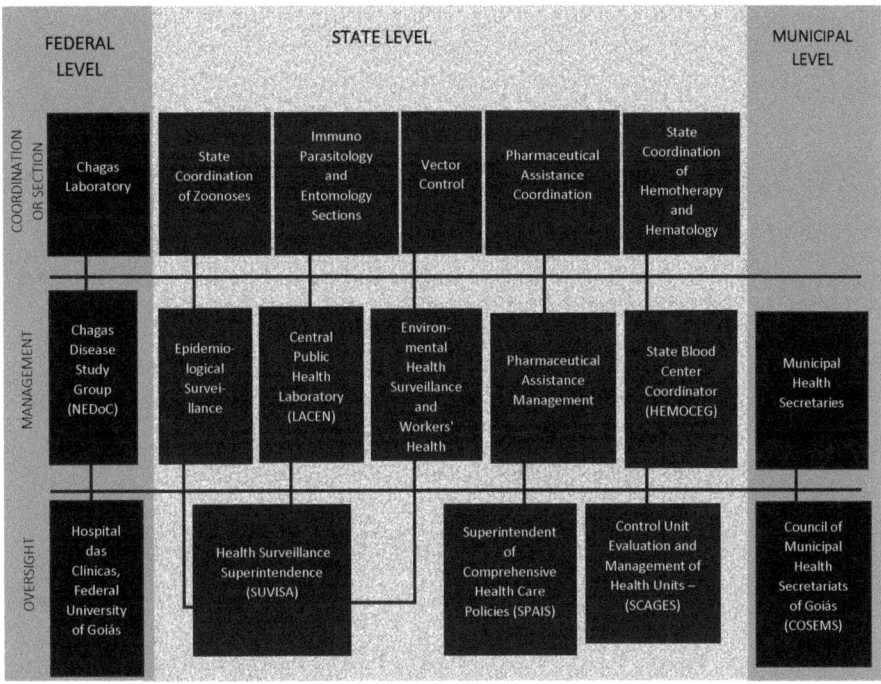

Figure 2. Main actors involved in the initiative to create the notification policy for chronic Chagas disease.

3.3. Implementation

The resolution approved by the State Department of Health went into effect on 6 May 2013, following the dissemination of the policy to regional health departments and municipalities. Implementation was carried out through the capacity building of professionals in the region and the technical support provided by the team responsible for the disease.

According to the experience of participants, there are ongoing limitations in the capacity to implement the policy in different areas. Human resources are considered the most critical point in the process due to the high turnover of health professionals, limited knowledge about the disease, and the lack of commitment from teams. However, all 18 state regional units, and their regional managers, and all 48 blood banks in the state (both private and public) were trained for notification in 2013. The state also promotes systematic training for Chagas disease, which includes training on the notification process. From 2017–2019, 960 health professionals, including doctors, nurses, and laboratory personnel, received this training in nine of the state's 18 regional units.

Another challenge in implementing the policy was obtaining support from managers and state agencies for monitoring of the notifications. Engagement of managers achieved in implementing the compulsory notification of chronic cases in the state was motivated by the mandatory nature described in the resolution. It was also motivated by increases in media dissemination of local cases and the alerts presented by technicians of the zoonosis team.

The goals outlined as a result of the implementation of the notification were framed in improving the access of patients with chronic Chagas to the public health system. Therefore, it was possible to establish parameters for the decentralization of care and monitoring of patients; train medical teams in diagnosis and treatment; consolidate the state network to deal with complications associated with the disease, and resume the vector control programs and entomological research. The state's annual health plan supports the financial sustainability of the program. The state has provided a budget for all activities related to notification since its implementation in 2013.

3.4. Evaluation

According to the opinions of the participants, the current notification of chronic cases of Chagas in the state is occurring systematically and has been quite consistent since 2014. The case investigation form has become a commonly used method for initiating laboratory diagnosis. There was a substantial increase in the reporting of chronic cases during the first 2 years of compulsory notification: from only 7 cases annually in 2013 (prior to full implementation), to 162 in the first year of the policy (2014), to 880 in 2015. Since then the reported cases have continued to increase by roughly 5%–10% each year, averaging 936 annually from 2015–2019.

However, it is important to improve communication processes with the municipalities and continuously train medical teams so that the entire notification system is effective and efficient. The steps of the current notification process described by the interviewees are shown in Figure 3.

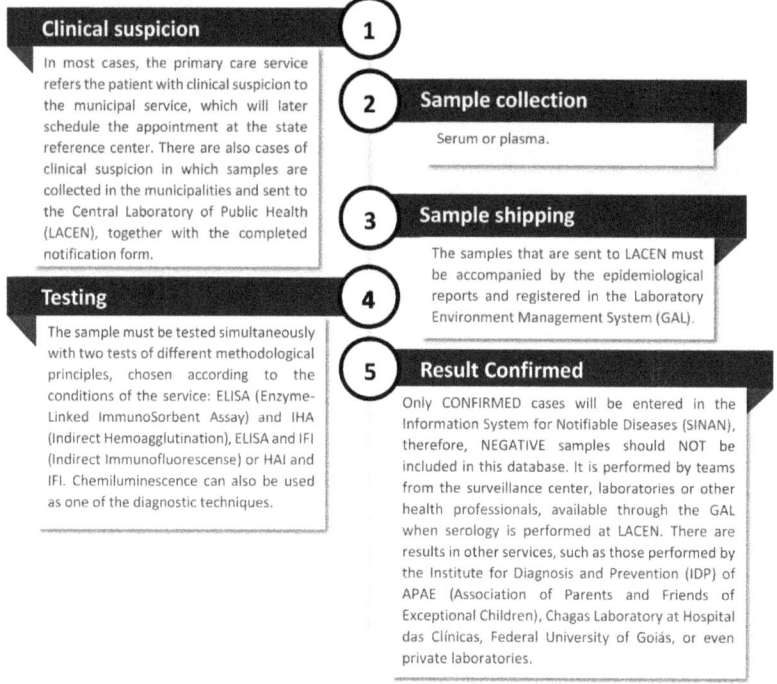

Figure 3. The current process of case notification of chronic Chagas disease in Goiás.

Only confirmed cases are entered into the SINAN (*Sistema de Informação de Agravos de Notificação*, or Information System for Notifiable Diseases). Therefore, negative samples are not included in this database. The notification is made by the core surveillance teams, by the laboratories or other health professionals, available through the Laboratory Environment Manager when the serology is performed at the Dr. Giovanni Cysneiros State Laboratory of Public Health. There are results in other services, such as those carried out by the Institute of Diagnosis and Prevention (IDP) of the Association of Parents and Friends of Special People (APAE, *Associação de Pais e Amigos dos Excepcionais*), the Chagas Laboratory at the Hospital of the Federal University of Goiás or even private laboratories.

4. Discussion

The lack of specific, complete and integrated information on the total number of people affected by Chagas disease frustrates the definition of public health response strategies ensuring adequate care for this population. For this reason, the creation and implementation of a public policy for notification of chronic cases in the state of Goiás is a strategic method for addressing the epidemiological silence of a highly neglected disease. Regionally, most epidemiological surveillance schemes for Chagas are limited to entomological surveillance, with or without seroepidemiological support [12,13]. In Goiás, the lack of information and activities to improve the care of people with Chagas led to the development of a specific public policy of notification. The obligation to report chronic cases thereby addresses a historical problem in the surveillance system of Goiás.

Public policies are the product of the government, but their construction is the result of a complex social interaction with the participation of various actors [14]. The stages in the design of a policy cycle correspond to a sequence of elements in the political-administrative process. They can be researched concerning its actors, their relationships, their resources, their political and social networks and their practices, typically found in each phase [15]. The main actors involved in the initiative identified several critical points that defined the initial context of the proposal, justifying the need for intervention. The cycle of neglect is fed by low visibility of people affected in the country, and limited knowledge by professionals and authorities about the disease. This culminates in the failure to report the disease and the lack of interest in preventive or control actions from some professionals and priority technical areas. The identification of chronic Chagas cases in public and private services leads to obtaining a more accurate snapshot of the population needing care, facilitating the implementation of services adapted to the needs of patients and appropriate, timely allocation of resources.

The guidelines for compulsory notification of diseases or conditions in the national surveillance system are usually generated and established by the Ministry of Health. However, states and municipalities are allowed to include other diseases or conditions, according to the local epidemiological reality. Goiás was the first state in Brazil to establish the obligation to report chronic Chagas disease. This important state challenge was supported by federal guidelines enabling the establishment of procedures for preparing a resolution with the support of state managers.

Notification of chronic Chagas disease has gained significant traction in Brazil following the adoption of the policy in Goiás. A resolution supporting notification SES/MG No. 6532 was enacted in the state of Minas Gerais in December 2018. In February 2020, an ordinance of the Brazilian Ministry of Health called for notification of chronic cases of Chagas disease throughout the national territory [16], which was updated in May 2020 [17]. This represents a significant opportunity to increase access to testing and treatment for over one million people [6] living with the disease in Brazil. The Goiás experience could serve as a guide for other states interested in strengthening local systems. Key lessons learned from the implementation of the notification of chronic Chagas disease in Goiás are shown in Figure 4.

According to local experience, the two biggest obstacles to implementation faced by the parties involved in the process were the lack of human resources and dissemination of the new guideline. Despite the recognized institutional capacity, technical knowledge, proactivity, commitment and dedication of the state technical team, these aspects continue to be significant challenges due to the high turnover of professionals at the municipal level. Clear articulation with partners from similar areas and the commitment of the technical Chagas program team have been essential to deal adequately with these implementation difficulties. Another permanent challenge for Goiás is assuring the quality of the data collected and its systematic analysis, as well as the ability to answer the training needs of health professionals addressing the mandatory notification of Chagas disease.

Guidelines	Surveillance	Health Services	Communication / visibility / work networks
a. Define key populations for the disease control process (for example, blood donors and pregnant women) b. Include Chagas serology in prenatal examinations ; c. Include mandatory investigation/ notification by a specific form by the patient's place of consultation when chronic Chagas is suspected; d. Immediately report reactive cases; e. Implement public policies for Chagas to improve clarity for providers and care for patients	a. Link collection and processing of samples for confirmation to an epidemiological investigation form ; b. Establish a Chagas Disease Surveillance Network; c. Conducting a Health Situation Analysis to establish whether the disease is a priority within the State and what actions are needed to address gaps	a. Include Chagas serology in prenatal examinations ; b. Improve the quality of access to the public health system for Chagas patients; c. Identify reference physicians who can offer guidance or answer questions from other clinicians; d. use telemedicine and other technologies; e. Develop preventive action strategies when new (acute) cases are identified f. Develop care strategies for identified chronic patients g. Monitor the children of women with Chagas disease.	a. Assure the commitment of technicians and managers throughout the process b. Establish a collaborative with the different actors in the health system, including universities; c. Establish committees or working groups to raise awareness of the importance of notification. d. Communicate the process to health technicians and the population before, during and after implementation.

Figure 4. Recommendations and lessons learned from the implementation of notification of chronic Chagas disease in Goiás.

A vital contribution to the design of the guideline was the definition of key populations. The inclusion of blood donors and pregnant women as priority surveillance populations for the disease control process contributed to the strengthening of the system.

The notification policy has a substantial impact on the visibility of people affected by Chagas disease and in the planning and execution of public health responses. Having consolidated information that describes the real distribution of the disease in the population, as well as the factors that determine the condition of neglect, allows development of tools to achieve better prevention and control actions, reactivating the Chagas state program as a whole [18].

Chagas disease is also reportable in six states in the United States. Although the main goal of this is to identify sources of local vector transmission, these states typically include reporting of chronic cases as well. As in the case of Goiás, compulsory notification has served to strengthen awareness among health professionals, although rates of diagnosed and treated patients remain very low [19]. This underscores the fact that reporting of Chagas and other neglected diseases needs to occur in conjunction with a variety of other complementary public health actions, such as capacity building, fortifying diagnostic capabilities, and providing information to at-risk communities.

The HIV/AIDS epidemic is another important example where a notification process played a key role. Initially, infection by the virus was identified exclusively in the clinical stage of the disease as acquired immunodeficiency syndrome (AIDS). The progress achieved in diagnosis and early treatment of the infection demonstrated the opportunity and importance of surveillance for cases of HIV infection, not being limited only to AIDS cases. Thus, several factors strengthened the increase in the number of people diagnosed, such as greater access to antiretroviral therapies (ART), the importance of starting treatment at an early stage, and the implementation of mother-to-child transmission prevention programs. In this context, the surveillance of HIV infection cases and the need for their notification became increasingly relevant [11].

In the effort to make Chagas disease more visible, regional and global initiatives are discussing and urging compulsory notification in the chronic phase, including the International Federation of Associations of People Affected by Chagas Disease (FINDECHAGAS) [20], and the Chagas Disease Clinical Research Platform [21]. Notification is a gateway to a surveillance system that should guarantee an opportunity to timely medical care and, ideally, social and mental health support for affected people [22]. It also reinforces and reactivates entomological surveillance and vector control activities.

Notification of chronic cases is an essential tool which, in conjunction with capacity building of healthcare personnel, availability of diagnosis and treatment in facilities accessible to affected people, implementation of simplified diagnostic processes, and development of safer, more efficacious treatments, can usher in the end to the neglect of Chagas disease.

Author Contributions: Conceptualization, A.M. and J.-C.C.; methodology, J.-C.C. and A.M.; software, M.P.C.; validation, L.d.R.S., F.A.d.S., and M.P.C.; formal analysis, J.-C.C.; investigation, L.d.R.S.; resources, C.F.; data curation, J.-C.C.; writing—original draft preparation, J.-C.C and A.M.; writing—review and editing, C.F.; visualization, M.P.C.; supervision, F.A.d.S.; project administration, A.M. All authors have read and agreed to the published version of the manuscript.

Funding: This research received no external funding.

Acknowledgments: Alejandro Luquetti-Universidade Federal de Goiás, UFG; Angélica Socorro do Nascimento Acioli-Biomédica-Coordenadora da Seção de Imunoparasitologia; Carolina Batista-Médicos Sem Fronteiras, Brasil; Daniella Carpaneda Machado-Médica Veterinária-Gestora de Recursos Naturais; Halim Antonio Girade-Secretaria de Estado da Saúde de Goiás; Huilma Alves Cardoso-Coordenação do Centro de Referência em Saúde do Trabalhador do Estado de Goiás; Marcelo Santalúcia-Centro Estadual de Referência em Medicina Integrativa e Complementar/CREMIC; Sergio Sosa-Estani-DNDi (Drugs for Neglected Diseases *initiative*); Sonaide Faria Ferreira Marques-Coordenação Estadual de Zoonoses da Secretaria de Estado da Saúde de Goiás; Tânia da Silva Vaz-Programas Especiais da Secretaria de Estado da Saúde de Goiás; Vitoria Ramos-Médicos Sem Fronteiras, Brasil; The Drugs for Neglected Diseases *initiative* (DNDi) appreciates the support of its donors, public and private, who have provided funding to DNDi since its creation in 2003. A complete list of DNDi donors can be found at http://www.dndi.org/donors/donors/

Conflicts of Interest: The authors declare no conflict of interest.

References

1. World Health Organization. *Working to Overcome the Global Impact of Neglected Tropical Diseases*; World Health Organization: Geneva, Switzerland, 2010.
2. Qian, M.; Zhou, X. Global burden on neglected tropical diseases. *Lancet Infect. Dis.* **2016**, *16*, 1113–1114. [CrossRef]
3. Ministry of Health of Brazil. National Mandatory Notification List [Internet]. Available online: http://portalms.saude.gov.br/vigilancia-em-saude/lista-nacional-de-notificacao-compulsoria (accessed on 17 July 2019).
4. Cardoso, C.S.; Ribeiro, A.L.P.; Oliveira, C.D.L.; Oliveira, L.C.; Ferreira, A.M.; Bierrenbach, A.L.; Silva, J.L.P.; Colosimo, E.A.; Ferreira, J.E.; Lee, T.-H.; et al. Beneficial effects of benznidazole in Chagas disease: NIH SaMi-Trop cohort study. *PLoS Neglected Trop. Dis.* **2018**, *12*, e0006814. [CrossRef] [PubMed]
5. Lee, B.; Bacon, K.; Bottazzi, M.; Hotez, P. Global economic burden of Chagas disease: A computational simulation model. *Lancet Infect. Dis.* **2013**, *13*, 342–348. [CrossRef]
6. World Health Organization. Chagas disease in Latin America: An epidemiological update based on 2010 estimates. *Wkly. Epidemiol. Rec.* 2015. Available online: https://www.who.int/wer/2015/wer9006.pdf?ua=1 (accessed on 20 June 2019).
7. Ferreira, I.; Silva, T. Elimination of Chagas disease transmission by Triatoma infestans in Brazil: A historical fact. *J. Braz. Soc. Trop. Med.* **2006**, *39*, 507–509. [CrossRef] [PubMed]
8. World Health Organization. Chagas disease, Brazil-Interruption of transmission. *Wkly. Epidemiol. Record* **2000**. Available online: https://apps.who.int/iris/bitstream/handle/10665/231149/WER7519_153-155.PDF (accessed on 20 June 2019).

9. Alves Moraes, C.; Ostermayer Luquetti, A.; Gonçalves Moraes, P.; Gonçalves de Moraes, C.; Elisabeth Campos Oliveira, D.; Chaves Oliveira, E. Proportional mortality ratio due to chagas disease is five times higher for the state of goias than the rest of brazil. *Rev. De Patol. Trop.* **2017**, *46*, 35. [CrossRef]
10. Saraiva, E. Introdução à teoria da política pública. In *Políticas Públicas Coletânea*; Saraiva, E., Ed.; Enap: Brasília, Brazil, 2006; Volume 2.
11. Organização Panamericana De Saúde (OPAS). *Vigilancia de la Infección por el VIH Basada en la Notificación de Casos: Recomendaciones para Mejorar y Fortalecer los Sistemas de Vigilancia del VIH*; OPS: Washington, DC, USA, 2012.
12. Dias, J. Controle da doença de Chagas. In *Clínica e Terapêutica da Doença de Chagas: Uma Abordagem para o Clínico Geral*; Editora Fiocruz: Rio de Janeiro, Brazil, 1997.
13. Dias, J. Problemas e possibilidades de participação comunitária no controle das grandes endemias no Brasil. *Cad. De Saúde Pública* **1998**, *14*, 19–37. [CrossRef]
14. Rua, M.G. Política pública: Conceitos básicos e achados empíricos. In *Políticas Públicas*; Rua, M.G., Ed.; IGEPP: Brasília, Brazil, 2013.
15. Howlett, M.; Ramesh, M.; Perl, A. *Politica Publica. Seus ciclos e subsistemas: Uma abordagem integral. Ed Campus*; Elsevier: Rio de Janeiro, Brazil, 2013.
16. Brazil. Portaria n° 264, de 17 de fevereiro de 2020. *Diário Oficial da União—Seção 1*, ISSN1 1677-7042. N° 35, quarta-feira, 19 de fevereiro de 2020. ISSN2 1677-7042.
17. Brazil. Portaria n° 1.061, de 18 de maio de 2020. *Diário Oficial da União—Seção 1*, ISSN 1677-7042. N° 102, sexta-feira, 29 de maio de 2020.
18. Dias, J. Vigilância epidemiológica contra Triatoma infestans. *Rev. Da Soc. Bras. De Med. Trop.* **1993**, *26*, 39–44.
19. Bennett, C.; Straily, A.; Haselow, D.; Weinstein, S.; Taffner, R.; Yaglom, H.; Komatsu, K.; Venkat, H.; Brown, C.; Byers, P.; et al. Chagas Disease Surveillance Activities-Seven States, 2017. *Mmwr Morb. Mortal. Wkly. Rep.* **2018**, *67*, 738–741. [CrossRef] [PubMed]
20. Coalizão Chagas. Las personas afectadas por Chagas de todo el mundo unen sus voces en un solo grito desde México [Internet]. 2019. Available online: http://www.coalicionchagas.org/news-article/-/asset_publisher/hJnt8AyJM2Af/content/las-personas-afectadas-por-chagas-de-todo-el-mundo-unen-sus-voces-en-un-solo-grito-desde-mexico (accessed on 17 July 2019).
21. DNDi. Carta de Santa Cruz [Internet]. 2019. Available online: http://bit.ly/carta-santa-cruz-por (accessed on 17 July 2019).
22. Dias, J. Vigilância epidemiológica em doença de Chagas. *Cadernos de Saúde Pública* **2000**, *16* (Suppl. 2), S43–S59. [CrossRef]

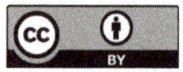

© 2020 by the authors. Licensee MDPI, Basel, Switzerland. This article is an open access article distributed under the terms and conditions of the Creative Commons Attribution (CC BY) license (http://creativecommons.org/licenses/by/4.0/).

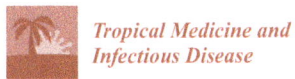

Article

Clinical, Cardiological and Serologic Follow-Up of Chagas Disease in Children and Adolescents from the Amazon Region, Brazil: Longitudinal Study

Ana Yecê das Neves Pinto [1,*], Vera da Costa Valente [1], Sebastião Aldo da Silva Valente [1], Tamires Anastácia Rodrigues Motta [2] and Ana Maria Revorêdo da Silva Ventura [1,2]

1. Instituto Evandro Chagas/Secretaria de Vigilância em Saúde/Ministério da Saúde-Brasil, Ananindeua 67030-000, Pará, Brazil; veravalente@iec.gov.br (V.d.C.V.); aldovalente@iec.gov.br (S.A.d.S.V.); ana_mariaventura@hotmail.com (A.M.R.d.S.V.)
2. Departamento de Saúde Integrada, Universidade do Estado do Pará, Belém 66050-540, Pará, Brazil; anastasia.motta@gmail.com
* Correspondence: ayece@iec.gov.br

Received: 15 June 2020; Accepted: 11 August 2020; Published: 31 August 2020

Abstract: Background: Outbreaks of Chagas disease (CD) by foodborne transmission is a problem related to deforestation, exposing people to triatomines infected by T. cruzi, in the Amazon region. Once involving long-time follow-up, the treatment efficacy of the CD during its acute phase is still unknown. The authors aim to describe the clinical and epidemiologic profile of children and adolescents with CD, as well as treatment and cardiac involvement during the follow-up. **Methods**: A descriptive cohort study was conducted from 1998 to 2013 among children and adolescents up to 18 years-old with confirmed diagnosis of CD. All participants met the criteria of CD in the acute phase. **Results**: A total of 126 outpatients were included and received treatment and follow-up examinations during a medium period of 10.9 years/person. Most of them (68.3%) had their diagnosis established during oral transmission outbreaks. The diagnostic method with the most positive results rate (80.9%) was the IgM class anti-*T. cruzi* antibody test as an acute phase marker, followed by the thick blood smears (60.8%). Acute myopericarditis was demonstrated in 18.2% of the patients, most of them with favorable evolution, though 2.4% (3/126) persisted with cardiac injury observed at the end point of the follow-up. **Conclusions**: Antibodies against *T. cruzi* persisted in 54.8% of sera from the patients without prognostic correlation with cardiac involvement. Precocious treatment can decrease potential cardiac complications and assure good treatment response, especially for inhabitants living in areas with difficult accessibility.

Keywords: Chagas disease; Cohort studies; Neglected diseases; *Trypanosoma cruzi*; Dynamic programming

1. Introduction

Since 1996, there has been an increase in the number of cases of Chagas disease (CD) in Brazil, especially in the states Pará and Amapá in the Brazilian Amazon. There, CD has shown different transmission patterns from other regions, with predominant presentation in focal recurrent and seasonal episodes affecting persons of the same family or neighbors, mainly by contaminated food. This emerging route of transmission has been the subject of innumerous epidemiological studies that added, over ten years, sufficient epidemiological evidence to explain some of these episodes as a consequence of accidental food contamination involving fruits ingested in natura under poor hygienic conditions [1].

In the past, data from most of the endemic areas of Chagas disease in Brazil recorded the acute phase of the disease as an inapparent form among children, on contrary of those cases occurred in the Amazon region [2,3]. In Pará state, the disease has peculiarities that are expressed as a very differentiated clinical entity of chronic disease with high morbidity. It is characterized by acute febrile syndrome, with manifestations of fever, chills, headache and myalgia and subcutaneous edema, in addition to reversible acute cardiac commitment, after treatment [4]. Chronic phase-type records of dilated cardiomyopathy are rare in the Amazon region [3].

For epidemiological surveillance, the precocious access to diagnosis is an important strategy regarding the precocious treatment. Nonspecific clinical features may be one of the reasons for low suspicion and late diagnosis [5–7]. This delay also is due to the low capacity of regional health professionals in including the patients into the diagnosis flows. In addition, since CD is inserted in a historical context of chronic illness, frequently the physician mis suspicion the febrile acute phase of the disease.

The description of CD related to all age groups will help the health professionals to increase knowledge about its morbidity profile, including cardiac complications, especially in the case of suspicious diagnosis, which will make a precocious diagnosis possible. In addition, the clinical descriptions of endemic areas of classical vector CD transmission no longer satisfy the unusual Amazonian epidemiology of this disease, requiring that the new descriptions be widely disseminated. In this sense, the objective is to characterize a historical cohort of children and adolescents under 18 years of age regarding their follow-up related to immediate and mediate treatment, until the outcome. The authors hope that a detailed description of the clinical profile of children and adolescents with CD here reported may be an useful tool as an evidence to strengthen the trainings of professionals in the management/diagnosis of suspected cases and thus, contribute to minimize the delay in diagnosis of this age group.

2. Materials and Methods

Study population: It consisted in a prospective historical cohort study of patients with acute CD phase, diagnosed since 1996. All participants were treated and followed up in the reference service for the follow-up of CD patients in the state of Pará, which operates according to the Clinical Protocols on Chagas Disease (PCDCha) and is located at the Unified Medical Care Service–Instituto Evandro Chagas (SOAMU/IEC). All patients included in the study were enrolled according to the ethical precepts of human research on a voluntary basis in accordance with their legal representatives. The project was approved by the research ethics committee of the IEC (ethical approval code n. 655.002) in accordance with the CD clinical protocol.

Procedures: All the participants met the criteria of acute phase: persons confirmed with clinical (signs and symptoms of febrile acute disease), epidemiological (another member of family or neighbor confirmed with CD) and with direct or indirect positive parasitological tests and/or a serologic reagent test with an acute phase marker (IgM against *T. cruzi*).

Data collection was carried out by analysis of medical records of the individuals eligible for the study. The following demographic data were evaluated: origin of the infection; likely transmission; contact with insect vectors; maternal prenatal history in children under two years of age; food history in children under two years of age; previous family history of Chagas disease; acute phase clinical data with information on the onset and interval time of the disease, initial disease suspicion, predominant signs and symptoms, coinfections, previous diseases, diagnostic results, nonspecific tests results and acute myocardial damage with emphasis on electrical conduction disorders.

Three probable modes of transmission were considered by the authors: Oral (or vectorial-oral) transmission—occurred during an outbreak of CD related to accidental ingestion of triatomines feces or even smashed triatomine in beverages. In these outbreaks the children and their family members had their diagnosis simultaneously made); vectorial transmission—children with history of contact with triatomine vectors; vertical transmission—children up to one years-old whose mother was also infected.

Two phases composed the temporal cohort data: one representing all eligible outpatients with acute phase of CD and a second including the same patients in a phase called follow-up after treatment corresponding to a medium period 10.5 years per person. (See Figure 1—design)

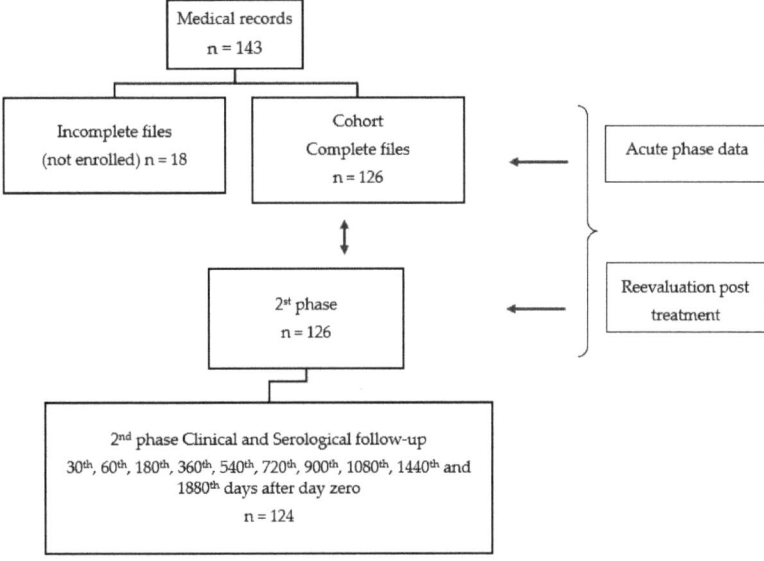

Figure 1. Study design.

The outcomes considered the following variables analyzed simultaneously: negative serologic conversion or persistence of IgG antibodies against *T. cruzi* with or without disease; persistence of IgG antibodies against *T. cruzi* with heart disease compatible changes in electrocardiogram or in echocardiogram compatible with CD (See Methods).

Laboratory evaluation: The patients underwent a blood count, parasitological (quantitative buffy coat (QBC®) or thick blood smear) and serologic tests, performed at the time of diagnosis or shortly before starting treatment and repeated sequentially after treatment, including thick blood smear, blood culture and serologic tests for the detection of anti-*T. cruzi* IgM and IgG antibodies.

Serologic techniques were carried out using the indirect hemagglutination assay (IHA) kit Hemacruzi, Biomérieux (qualitative assay) and the indirect immunofluorescence assay (IIF)-kit Imunocruzi, Biomérieux for titration (quantitative assay) of IgM and IgG classes of immunoglobulins. For the latter, anti-human IgM and IgG labeled with fluorescein (BIOLAB, Brazil) were used. For IHA, a titer of 1:40 was tested and for IIF, sera dilutions from 1:40 up to 1:1280 were tested. The reference value for both tests was a nonreagent result at the 1:40 or less dilution.

The serologic follow-up post treatment was analyzed cumulatively according to individual evaluations. These were performed according to service protocols on the first day of treatment (day zero) and sequentially on the 30th, 60th, 180th, 360th, 540th, 720th, 900th, 1080th, 1440th and 1880th day after day zero.

The evaluation also included blood analysis and platelet measures. Hemoglobin rate according to age and gender determined anemia (Hb < 11 g% in children from 6 months up 9 years of age; <12 g% in female adolescents; <13 g% in male adolescents).

The normal reference values to the leucocyte counts ranged from 5000 to 10,000 /mm^3. Values below or above this range were defined as leukopenia and leukocytosis. The normal reference values for platelet levels ranged from 150,000 to 300,000 /mm^3. The values below or above this range defined thrombocytopenia or thrombocytosis.

For the clinical classifications of cardiac involvement levels during the acute phase, only the results of electrocardiograms (EKG) and echocardiograms from this phase were evaluated. The echocardiograms were used only to classify the acute stage, but not for the follow-up. To this analysis, the parameters already described in Amazonian populations [5] were considered:

(1) Severe cardiac involvement: heart failure caused by chagasic infection as evidenced by echocardiogram results demonstrating severe myopericarditis with pericardial effusion;
(2) Moderate cardiac involvement: myocarditis accompanied by sinus tachycardia or other arrhythmias with pericarditis and pericardial effusion;
(3) Mild cardiac involvement: myocarditis accompanied by sinus tachycardia or other simple conduction disorders.

The outcomes were classified by the analysis of three parameters: (a) negative serologic conversion, for those with a sequence of three negative serologic antibodies test in two different methods; (b) undefined, for those with loss of serologic follow-up; (c) persistence of IgG antibodies against *T. cruzi* without evidence of disease; (d) persistence of IgG antibodies against *T. cruzi* with cardiac disease compatible with CD.

Analysis: To evaluate the serologic follow-up time, the mean follow-up time per person-year was calculated, considering the year of inclusion into the study, subtracted from the most recent evaluation year (2013) and divided by the number of years elapsed between primary inclusion (1998) through the most recent evaluation (e.g., 2013). Thus, from these calculations, the mean follow-up time per year-person after treatment was 10.9 years.

The geometric means of anti-*T. cruzi* IgG antibody titers as measured by IIF were compared on two different points of time, based on day zero as the start of treatment. Therefore, the measurements were compared on days zero and 720th or two years after treatment and on days zero and 1800th or five years after treatment, using analysis of variance (ANOVA) test, using 5% as the significance level.

3. Results

3.1. Demographic Data, Origin and Spatial Distribution

A total of 126 children and adolescents from 0 up to 18 years of age treated during the acute phase of the disease were evaluated from 1998 to 2013. The origin of infection were located in both urban and rural municipal areas of Pará and one city of Amapá state (Table 1, Figure 2).

Table 1. Demographic and epidemiological data from patients with Chagas disease from Amazon region, Brazil.

Epidemiological Data	Frequency	%
Age (years)		
0–2	4	3.2
3–7	20	15.9
8–11	40	31.8
12–17	62	49.2
Gender		
Female	46	36.6
Male	80	63.4
Origin		
Pará State regions		
Baixo Amazonas	1	0.8
Marajó Island	26	20.8
Metropolitan area of Belém	52	41.2
Northeast	41	32.5
Southeast	2	1.6
Amapá State		
Santana	4	3.2

Table 1. *Cont.*

Epidemiological Data	Frequency	%
Transmission form		
Oral	86	68.3
Vectorial	19	15.1
Vertical	2	1.6
Undefined	19	15.1
Outbreak		
Yes	90	71.4
No	35	27.8
Undefined	1	0.8

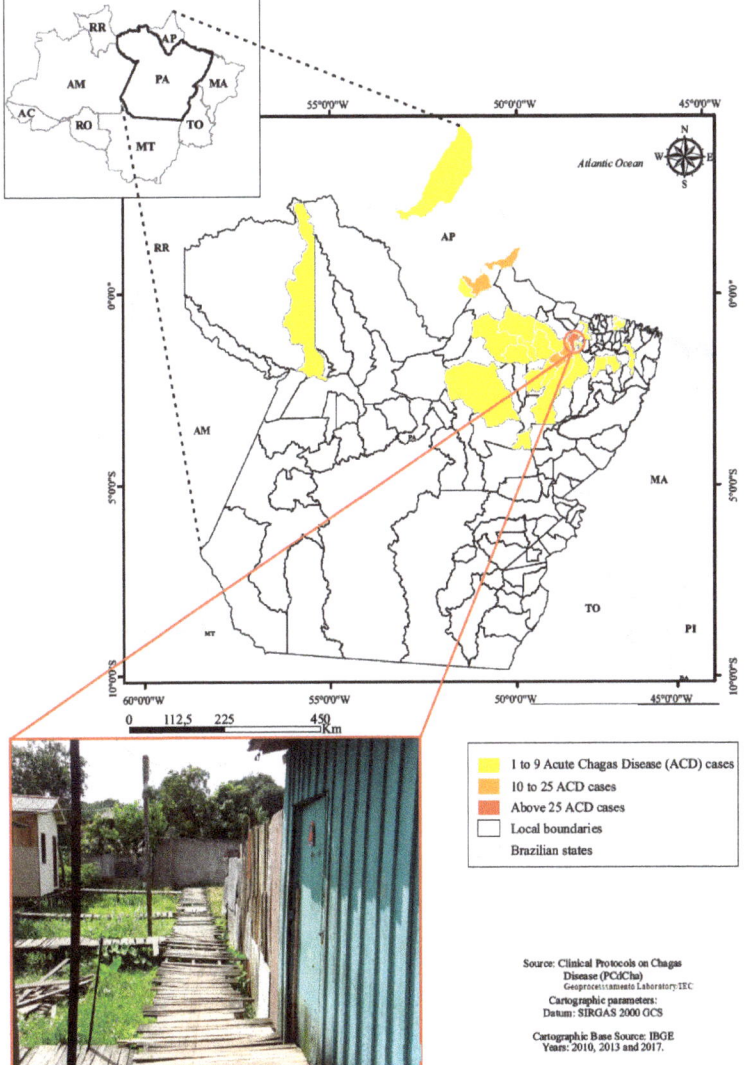

Figure 2. Residence location of children and adolescents with acute Chagas disease, Belém, Pará, Amazon region, Brazil.

The mean follow-up time per person-year after treatment was 10.9 years. The mean period of illness from the onset of symptoms to the diagnosis was 33.2 days.

3.2. Clinical Features

The most frequent clinical manifestations among the participants were acute febrile syndrome in 92.8% and cardiac involvement in 16.1% (Table 2).

Table 2. Main clinical manifestations in young patients with Chagas disease.

Clinical Manifestations	Frequency	%	Clinical Manifestations	Frequency	%
Fever	117	92.8	Hepatomegaly	34	26.9
Headache	74	58.7	Chills	27	21.4
Pallor	64	50.8	Caught	24	19.0
Myalgia	56	44.4	Splenomegaly	24	19.0
Abdominal pain	54	42.8	Exanthema	20	15.9
Edema of face	53	42.1	Edema of lower limbs	19	15.1
Adenopathy	49	38.9	Chest pain	13	10.3
Dyspnea	45	35.7	Palpitations	13	10.3
Arthralgia	44	34.9	Nodules in lower limbs	4	3.2
Diarrhea	34	26.9	Inoculation lesion	4	3.2

Direct parasitological examinations revealed a positivity rate of 60.8% by the thick blood smears and 54.9% by the QBC®method. The method with most high positivity rate was the IgM class of anti-*T. cruzi* antibodies test as an acute phase marker (80.9%) (Figure 3). Among patients with IgM tests nonreagent (24/126), all of them had parasitological test positive/reagent and/or serologic test IgG positive added to a clinical signs of the disease.

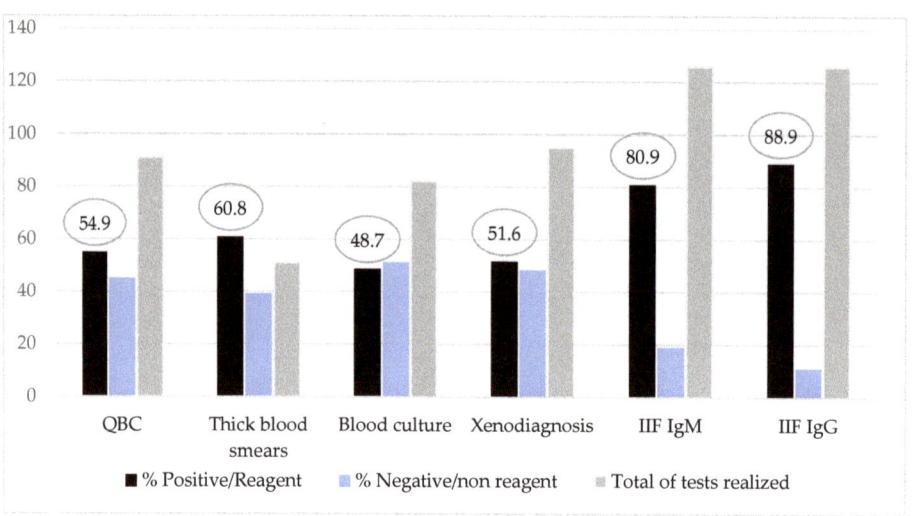

Figure 3. Diagnostic methods results rate from children and adolescents with Chagas disease.

Anemia with hemoglobin values of 7.6 mg/dL was the most frequent finding among hematological abnormalities (Table 3).

3.3. Acute Phase Cardiac Involvement

Among 88 patients who performed a complete evaluation with at least one of the two cardiac exams, i.e., EKG or echocardiogram, 18.2% (16/88) revealed some cardiac involvement and were classified according to clinical and electro- or echocardiographic results.

Table 3. Counts of blood cells according with age in young patients with Chagas disease before treatment.

Hematological Analysis	6–23 Months	2–6 y	7–9 y	≥10 y (Female)	≥10 y (Male)	Total N	%
Anemia	6	11	11	14	20	62	49.2
Reference hemoglobin concentration rate	2	6	6	3	9	25	19.8
Reference leukocytes count	3	10	15	11	27	66	52.3
Leukocytosis	5	6		2	1	14	11.1
Leukopenia		1	2	3	1	7	5.5
Reference platelets count	3	7	9	9	20	48	38.1
Thrombocytosis	5	8	4	4	7	28	22.2
Thrombocytopenia		2	1		1	4	3.2

In 52.9% of the patients, the resting electrocardiogram showed a normal result during the acute phase. Among those with altered exams, there was a higher frequency of diffuse repolarization and sinusal tachycardia (Table 4). On those submitted to echocardiogram, we observed 18.9% (16/88) with pericardial effusion, of whom 75.0% (12/16) had severe, 18.8% (3/16) mild and 6.2% (1/16) moderate cardiac involvement.

Table 4. Electrocardiographic abnormalities of children patients with Chagas disease before treatment.

Electrocardiogram	N	%
Normal	52	59.1
Abnormal	36	40.9
Diffuse repolarization abnormalities	10	27.8
Sinusal tachycardia	6	16.7
Conduction disturbances	3	8.3
Sinusal arrhythmia	2	5.5
Incomplete right bundle branch block	2	5.5
Block in the superior division of the left branch	2	5.5
Bradycardia sinusal	1	2.8
Complete left bundle branch block	1	2.8
First degree atrio ventricular block	1	2.8

3.4. Response to Treatment, Adverse Effects and Serologic Follow-Up after Treatment

Once the children were diagnosed, they were immediately treated within a medium period of 20.8 h, with a minimum of 2 h and maximum of 72 h. A total of 123 patients (97.6%) were treated with benznidazole and one was treated with nifurtimox, due to severe benznidazole adverse effect (described as follow). The study revealed that 94.3% of the patients (117/124) received treatment with drugs during 50 or more days, while only 5.6% (7/124) for less than 49 days. Among those who were treated for less than 49 days, five of them did so for at least 30 days and two just for one day. Those two children that have incomplete treatment were disregarded in this analysis. Adverse reactions occurred in 20.2% (25/124) of the patients consisting of dermatologic alterations (72%); hair loss (3%); gastric disturbances and insomnia (2%) as principal findings. Dermatological alterations included: maculopapular rash, urticaria, morbilliform exanthema and angioneurotic edema (Figure 4).

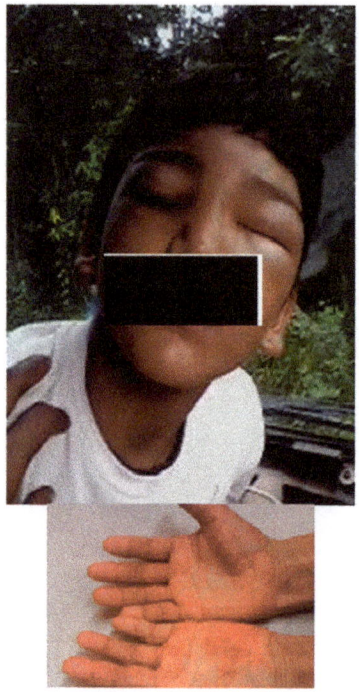

Figure 4. Face angioedema and maculopapular rush in hands post treatment with benznidazole, in two patients.

4. Clinical Follow-Up According to Serologic and Cardiac Evaluation

Throughout the serologic follow-up, the geometric means of antibody titers after treatment declined in medians of up to three titles (Figure 5).

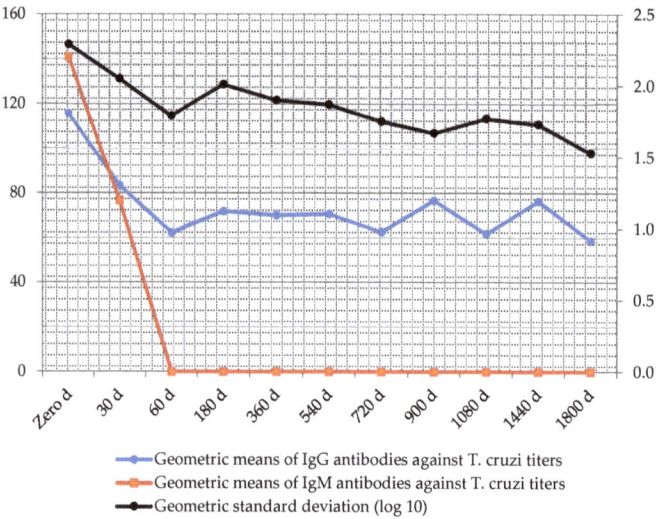

Figure 5. Follow-up geometric means of IgM and IgG antibody titers against *T. cruzi*, after treatment with antichagasic drugs measured by immunofluorescence absorbent tests.

According to the outcome evaluations which included cardiac exams and serologic tests before and after treatment until the end point, 54.8% of the patients demonstrated sustained reactive IgG antibody titers (low titers) without evidence of cardiac disease after the mean period of 10.9 person–years of follow-up (Table 5). See definitions in Methods.

Table 5. Evolution observed in the end point post treatment of patients with Chagas disease.

Evolution after Treatment	Frequency	%
Sustained nonreactive serologic tests	21	16.7
Persistence of IgG antibodies against *T. cruzi* without evidence of cardiac disease	69	54.8
Persistence of IgG antibodies against *T. cruzi* with evidence of cardiac injury	3	2.4
Undefined	33	26.2
Total	126	100

5. Discussion

In this observational study of monitoring patients over a period of 15 years, the conglomeration of patients in family outbreaks suggested oral transmission of 71.42%. In Brazil, there were 112 outbreaks in conglomerates between 2005 and 2013, with ingestion of contaminated foods as the most frequent form of transmission. However, more than 20% of the patients had no transmission information form registered, with 87.5% of them in the Pará state, due to failures of timely outbreak investigations [8].

Despite the smallest proportion of vector transmission (6.4%) in Brazil, persistence of focal points was observed, and entomological surveillance has been strengthened annually [8]. The national seroprevalence survey for the evaluation of CD control in Brazil conducted between 2001 and 2008 reported an infection prevalence of 0.03% among children under five years of age, in the majority suggesting vertical transmission due to maternal positive results and in the others indicating possible vectorial transmission [9,10]. In our sample, vector transmission was the second most frequent mode, as 71.4% of children and adolescents were infected during outbreaks with evidence of food transmission.

There were predominant manifestations of prolonged febrile syndrome, including the main triad of fever (92.85%), headache (58.73%) and cutaneous pallor (50.79%). Rassi & Ferreira (1971) reported fever as the main general manifestation, followed by ganglionic hypertrophy and subcutaneous edema in the same proportion of 45.94% in all their patients with a mean age of 12.1 years [11]. Pinto et al. (2007) corroborated that febrile syndrome is the principal clinical feature in 95% of patients with severe ACD, followed by dyspnea (75%) and asthenia (65%), in addition to other signs and symptoms, although the mean age of these patients was 46.7 years [12]. Shikanai-Yasuda et al. (1990) also registered a high frequency of fever (91.7%), lymph node enlargement (70.8%), hepatomegaly (66.7%), splenomegaly (41.7%), lower limb edema or generalized edema (62.5%), cutaneous rash (12.5%), cough (8.3%) and signs of congestive heart failure (16.7%) [13].

In patients previously studied in the Amazon region, the search for IgM and IgG antibody titers was essential for diagnosis in patients with prolonged disease because in these cases, the individual diagnosis was delayed, reducing the chance of parasite detection in the peripheral blood (5). In the series studied, the most effective tests to detect the infection were the serologic methods IgM and IgG against *T. cruzi* measured by IIF (80.9% and 88.9%), followed by parasitological methods thick blood smears (60.8%) and QBC®method (54.9%). This result strengths the recommended strategies of the Brazilian Chagas consensus about simultaneous serologic and parasitological procedures in suspected cases.

Anemia occurred in almost half (49.2%) of the patients, with a minimum value of hemoglobin concentration of 7.0 g% and a maximum of 15.0 g%, with a mean of 10.7 g%, which is below the reference value. Leukometry was on reference limits and therefore more frequently found than the registers from another outbreak (37.5%) of ACD in urban areas described by Shikanai-Yasuda et al. (1990) [13]. Thrombocytosis was frequently found, both in patients from this sample as from other series [5].

Among those who underwent EKG examination during the acute phase 59.1% did not have electrocardiographic abnormalities. However, among those with alterations, the main findings were diffuse repolarization abnormalities in 27.8% of patients, followed by sinus tachycardia (16.7%). Comparatively, in the study by Noya et al. (2010) that included 77 children during an acute phase outbreak in Venezuelan schoolchildren, the incidence of alterations was 69.7%. The abnormalities found in 40.9% were lower than those reported by Noya et al. (2010) in an outbreak of ACD [14].

In our study, we found diffuse repolarization abnormalities (27.8%) and sinus tachycardia (16.7%), which is also different from the study by Noya et al. (2010), whose main changes were T and P wave segments (37.8%) and arrhythmias (32%). Additionally, in our series, sinus tachycardia proved to be a signal during physical examination as suggestive of suspected ACD.

Another study made in the Amazon region including adults and children observed 52.3% of electrocardiographic changes, which was three times higher than the frequency in the children of this sample. Comparatively, the main electrocardiographic findings among adults were diffuse ventricular repolarization abnormalities (DVRA) (43.3%) and low voltage of the QRS axis (15.6%), while in the children studied, the findings were DVRA and sinus tachycardia [15].

Negative serum conversion is a marker used in follow-up studies after treatment. Although controversial, anti-*T. cruzi* IgG antibodies persistence at low levels in serial evaluations is used as a marker of cure. In Argentina, for example, 90% of children who completed treatment in 60 days had a persistent decrease or disappearance of specific anti-*T. cruzi* antibodies [16]. Corroborating the Argentine study, the Brazilian series studied showed an excellent response to treatment considering the established clinical cure criteria, especially the complete resolution of the symptoms and the persistent decrease in titration of IgG antibodies against *T. cruzi*. Negative seroconversion was observed at a lower frequency. When compared to the Argentine study, the authors questioned negative seroconversion as a potential cure marker and propose the PCR methodology in view to improve the cure rates most faithful [17].

Currently, only two drugs have demonstrated efficacy for the treatment of CD: nifurtimox, a nitrofuran derivative and benznidazole, a nitroimidazole derivative. Benznidazole is well tolerated among children, being less susceptible to adverse effects than adults and tolerating higher doses [18–20]. The most frequent adverse reactions in the studied group were dermatological alterations in 14.27% of them. Compared to the study by Altcheh et al. (2011), these adverse reactions were much less frequent than in the 71% of the patients in the age range between 10 days and 19 years of age. The main adverse reactions to the specific drug in Argentina consisted of dermatological complaints, such as skin rash, eczema, pruritus, polymorphic erythema and urticaria (16). In the Brazilian series, clinical follow-up showed that 54.8% had positive serologies without signals of disease; 16.7% were considered cured for having negative sustained serologic conversion in serial evaluations and only 2.4% were considered to have mild chronic cardiopathy.

Finally, it was possible to identify that the initial clinical manifestation in children and adolescents varies from febrile syndrome to complex cases of acute myopericarditis. Among those who had cardiac involvement, severe acute myocarditis affected 18.8% of them with faster resolution after immediate specific treatment. When comparing the clinical manifestation of the disease in children and adults, it is evident that in both, febrile syndrome was the most frequent manifestation. Second, dyspnea and asthenia are frequent manifestations in adults, while pallor and headaches are predominant in children and youth. In children, therefore, the presumed diagnosis of chagasic etiology is mandatory in those with prolonged fever or acute myocarditis. Anemia was the most frequent nonspecific laboratory abnormalities in children and adolescents.

We are in debt with the affected people in search for diagnostic tools that could access the cure rates most faithful, especially in those exposed to vertical transmission. The decrease in antibodies IgG against *T. cruzi* titers during the mean follow-up period of 10.5 years, after treatment and maintenance of those in lower titers confers antiparasitic immune memory persistence, which could suggest low potential evolution to chronic phase of the disease, after treatment with drugs received during the acute phase.

Author Contributions: Conceptualization A.Y.d.N.P. and A.M.R.d.S.V.; data curation A.Y.d.N.P., V.d.C.V., S.A.d.S.V. and A.M.R.d.S.V.; formal analysis, V.d.C.V. and A.Y.d.N.P.; funding acquisition V.d.C.V. and S.A.d.S.V.; investigation A.Y.d.N.P., S.A.d.S.V. and T.A.R.M.; visualization methodology S.A.d.S.V., V.d.C.V. and A.M.R.d.S.V.; supervision A.Y.d.N.P.; validation T.A.R.M.; visualization, V.d.C.V.; writing—original draft preparation, A.Y.d.N.P. and T.A.R.M.; writing—original draft, A.Y.d.N.P. and T.A.R.M.; writing—review & editing A.Y.d.N.P. and A.M.R.d.S.V. All authors have read and agreed to the published version of the manuscript.

Funding: This research was supported by Instituto Evandro Chagas (IEC)/Secretaria de Vigilância em Saúde/ Ministério da Saúde do Brasil.

Acknowledgments: We thank to all researcher technicians from SOAMU and from the Pathology and Chagas disease laboratories of the Evandro Chagas Institute. To Rilciane Maria dos Reis Ribeiro, Md. To Martin Johannes Eink for English revisions.

Conflicts of Interest: The authors declare no conflict of interest.

References

1. Panamerican Health Organization (PAHO/WHO). *Guide to Surveillance, Prevention, Control and Clinical Management of Acute Chagas Disease Transmitted by Food*; Technical Manuals Series, 12; PAHO: Rio de Janeiro, Brazil, 2009; p. 92. (In Brazilian)
2. Valente, S.A.D.S.; da Costa Valente, V.; das Neves Pinto, A.Y.; de Jesus Barbosa César, M.; dos Santos, M.P.; Miranda, C.O.S.; Cuervo, P.; Fernandes, O. Analysis of an acute Chagas disease outbreak in the Brazilian Amazon: Human cases, triatomines, reservoir mammals and parasites. *Trans. R. Soc. Trop. Med. Hyg.* **2009**, *103*, 291–297. [CrossRef]
3. Pinto, A.Y.D.N.; Valente, V.D.C.; Coura, J.R.; Valente, S.A.D.S.; Junqueira, A.C.V.; Santos, L.C.; De Macedo, R.C. Clinical Follow-Up of Responses to Treatment with Benznidazol in Amazon: A Cohort Study of Acute Chagas Disease. *PLoS ONE* **2013**, *8*, e64450. [CrossRef]
4. Pinto, A.Y.N. American Trypanosomiasis. In *Red Book:2018 Report of the Committee in Infectious Disease*, 31th ed.; Kimberlin, D.W., Brady, M.T., Jackson, M.A., Long, S.S., Eds.; American Academy of Pediatrics: Itasca, IL, USA, 2018; Volume I, pp. 826–829.
5. Pinto, A.Y.N.; Valente, S.A.S.; Valente, V.C.; Ferreira, A.R., Jr.; Coura, J.R. Acute phase of Chagas disease in the Amazon: Brazilian study of 233 cases from Pará, Amapá and Maranhão observed between 1988 and 2005. *Rev. Soc. Bras. Med. Trop.* **2008**, *41*, 602–614. [CrossRef] [PubMed]
6. Pinto, A.Y.N.; Valente, S.A.S.; Valente, V.C. Emerging acute Chagas disease in Amazonian Brazil: Case reports with serious cardiac involvement. *Braz. J. Infect. Dis.* **2004**, *8*, 458–464. [CrossRef] [PubMed]
7. de Barros Moreira Beltrão, H.; de Paula Cerroni, M.; de Freitas, D.R.C.; das Neves Pinto, A.Y.; da Costa Valente, V.; Valente, S.A.; Costa, E.D.G.; Sobel, J. Investigation of two outbreaks of suspected oral transmission of acute Chagas disease in the Amazon region, Pará State, Brazil, in 2007. *Trop. Doct.* **2009**, *39*, 231–232. [CrossRef] [PubMed]
8. Secretaria de Vigilância em Saúde. *Ministério da Saúde Brasil. Boletim Epidemiológico Doença de Chagas Aguda e Distribuição Espacial dos triatomíneos de Importância Epidemiológica, Brasil 2012 a 2016*; MS: Brasília, Brazil, 2019; Volume 50, p. 10.
9. Ostermayer, A.L.; Passos, A.D.C.; Silveira, A.C.; Ferreira, A.W.; Macedo, W.; Prata, A.R. National seroprevalence survey evaluation of the control of Chagas disease in Brazil (2001–2008). *Rev. Soc. Bras. Med. Trop.* **2011**, *44*, 108–121. [CrossRef] [PubMed]
10. Dias, J.C.P.; Ramos, N.A., Jr.; Gontijo, E.D.; Luquetti, A.; Shikanani-Yasuda, M.A.; Coura, J.R. II Consenso brasileiro em doença de Chagas, 2015. *Epidemiologia e Serviços de Saúde* **2016**, *25*, 7–86. [CrossRef] [PubMed]
11. Rassi, A.; Ferreira, H.O. Attempts of specific treatment of the acute stage of Chagas' disease with nitrofurans in prolonged schemes. *Rev. Soc. Bras. Med. Trop.* **1971**, *5*, 235–262. [CrossRef]
12. Pinto, A.Y.N.; Farias, J.R.; Marçal, A.S.; Galucio, S.; Costi, R.R.; Valente, V.C. Severe acute Chagas disease in the Amazon indigenous Brazilian. Available online: http://scielo.iec.gov.br/pdf/rpm/v21n2/v21n2a02.pdf (accessed on 12 August 2020).
13. Shikanai-Yasuda, M.A.; Lopes, M.H.; Tolezano, J.E.; Umezawa, E.; Amato, V.N.; Barreto, A.C.; Higaki, Y.; Moreira, A.A.; Funayama, G.; Barone, A.A. Acute Chagas' disease: Transmission routes, clinical aspects and response to specific therapy in diagnosed cases in an urban center. *Rev. Inst. Med. Trop.* **1990**, *32*, 16–27. [CrossRef] [PubMed]

14. Alarcón de Noya, B.; Díaz-Bello, Z.; Colmenares, C.; Ruiz-Guevara, R.; Mauriello, L.; Zavala-Jaspe, R.; Suarez, J.A.; Abate, T.; Naranjo, L.; Paiva, M.; et al. Large Urban Outbreak of Orally Acquired Acute Chagas Disease at a School in Caracas, Venezuela. *J. Infect. Dis.* **2010**, *201*, 1308–1315. [CrossRef] [PubMed]
15. Pinto, A.Y.N.; Ferreira, S.M.A.G.; Valente, S.A.S.; Valente, V.C.; Ferreira, A.G., Jr. Electrocardiographic changes during and after treatment with benznidazole in acute stage of Chagas disease indigenous to the brazilian Amazon. *Revista Pan-Amazônica de Saúde* **2010**, *1*, 67–76.
16. Altcheh, J.; Moscatelli, G.; Moroni, S.; Garcia-Bournissen Freilij, H. Adverse events after the use of benznidazole in infants and children with Chagas disease. *Pediatrics* **2011**, *127*, e212–e218. [CrossRef] [PubMed]
17. Meymandi, S.; Hernandez, S.; Park, S.; Sanchez, D.R.; Forsyth, C. Treatment of Chagas Disease in the United States. *Curr. Treat. Options Infect. Dis.* **2018**, *10*, 373–388. [CrossRef] [PubMed]
18. Machado-de-Assis, G.F.; Diniz, G.A.; Montoya, R.A.; Dias, J.C.P.; Coura, J.R.; Machado-Coelho, G.L.L.; Albajar-Viñas, P.; Torres, R.M.; Lana, M.D. A serological, parasitological and clinical evaluation of untreated Chagas disease patients and those treated with benznidazole before and thirteen years after intervention. *Memórias do Instituto Oswaldo Cruz* **2013**, *108*, 873–880. [CrossRef] [PubMed]
19. Morillo, C.; Marin-Neto, J.A.; Avezum, A.; Sosa-Estani, S.; Rosas, F.; Villena, E.; Quiroz, R.; Bonilla, R.; Britto, C.; Guhl, F.; et al. Benefit Investigators. Randomized trial of benznidazole for chronic Chagas' cardiomyopathy. *N. Engl. J. Med.* **2015**, *373*, 1295–1306. [CrossRef] [PubMed]
20. Carlier, Y.; Torrico, F.; Russomando, G.; Luquetti, A.; Freilji, H.; Albajar Vinas, P. Congenital Chagas disease: Recommendations for diagnosis, treatment and control of newborns, siblings and pregnant women. *PLoS Negl. Trop. Dis.* **2011**, *5*, e250. [CrossRef] [PubMed]

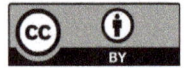

© 2020 by the authors. Licensee MDPI, Basel, Switzerland. This article is an open access article distributed under the terms and conditions of the Creative Commons Attribution (CC BY) license (http://creativecommons.org/licenses/by/4.0/).

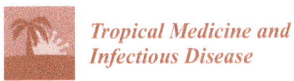 *Tropical Medicine and Infectious Disease*

Article

Progression Rate from the Indeterminate Form to the Cardiac Form in Patients with Chronic Chagas Disease: Twenty-Two-Year Follow-Up in a Brazilian Urban Cohort

Alejandro Marcel Hasslocher-Moreno *, Sergio Salles Xavier, Roberto Magalhães Saraiva, Luiz Henrique Conde Sangenis, Marcelo Teixeira de Holanda, Henrique Horta Veloso, Andrea Rodrigues da Costa, Fernanda de Souza Nogueira Sardinha Mendes, Pedro Emmanuel Alvarenga Americano do Brasil, Gilberto Marcelo Sperandio da Silva, Mauro Felippe Felix Mediano and Andrea Silvestre de Sousa

Evandro Chagas National Institute of Infectious Disease, Oswaldo Cruz Foundation, Rio de Janeiro 21040-900, Brazil; sergio.xavier@ini.fiocruz.br (S.S.X.); roberto.saraiva@ini.fiocruz.br (R.M.S.); luiz.sangenis@ini.fiocruz.br (L.H.C.S.); marcelo.holanda@ini.fiocruz.br (M.T.d.H.); henrique.veloso@ini.com.fiocruz (H.H.V.); andrea.costa@ini.fiocruz.br (A.R.d.C.); fernanda.sardinha@ini.fiocruz.br (F.d.S.N.S.M.); pedro.brasil@ini.fiocruz.br (P.E.A.A.d.B.); gilberto.silva@ini.fiocruz.br (G.M.S.d.S.); mauro.mediano@ini.fiocruz.br (M.F.F.M.); andrea.silvestre@ini.fiocruz.br (A.S.d.S.)
* Correspondence: alejandro.hasslocher@ini.fiocruz.br

Received: 7 April 2020; Accepted: 9 May 2020; Published: 12 May 2020

Abstract: Most patients with chronic Chagas disease (CD) present the indeterminate form and are at risk to develop the cardiac form. However, the actual rate of progression to the cardiac form is still unknown. Methods: In total, 550 patients with the indeterminate CD form were followed by means of annual electrocardiogram at our outpatient clinic. The studied endpoint was progression to cardiac form defined by the appearance of electrocardiographic changes typical of CD. The progression rate was calculated as the cumulative progression rate and the incidence progression rate per 100 patient years. Results: Thirty-seven patients progressed to the CD cardiac form within a mean of 73 ± 48 months of follow-up, which resulted in a 6.9% cumulative progression rate and incidence rate of 1.48 cases/100 patient years. Patients who progressed were older (mean age 47.8 ± 12.2 years), had a higher prevalence of associated heart diseases ($p < 0.0001$), positive xenodiagnosis ($p = 0.007$), and were born in the most endemic Brazilian states ($p = 0.018$). Previous co-morbidities remained the only variable associated with CD progression after multivariate Cox proportional hazards regression analysis ($p = 0.002$). Conclusion: The progression rate to chronic CD cardiac form is low and inferior to rates previously reported in other studies.

Keywords: Chagas disease; heart disease; electrocardiogram; disease progression

1. Introduction

Chagas disease (CD) is considered a neglected tropical disease by the World Health Organization, with an estimated 8 million people infected worldwide [1]. As a result of globalization, cases are no longer restricted to Latin America and this new paradigm is a new challenge to be overcome [2]. Control programs for vectorial and transfusional transmission of CD, developed in the 1980s, significantly decreased transmission. However, surveillance challenges remain due to new outbreaks of oral transmission in endemic countries [3] and to the possibility of vertical transmission, even in nonendemic areas [4]. The urbanization of the disease expanded access to healthcare services in endemic and non-endemic countries, changing their epidemiological profile, and together with CD control programs, led to an increase in the age range of patients [5]. Integrated surveillance and healthcare actions currently target the large number of patients already infected with *Trypanosoma cruzi* [6], a significant portion of whom may develop chronic Chagas heart disease (CHD), a major determinant of morbidity and mortality [7]. Studies on the indeterminate chronic form (ICF) of CD are usually cross-sectional, most of which were performed in rural areas and were only aimed at describing its prevalence, and rarely have prospective designs. Approximately 50% of the infected people have ICF, which is characterized by low morbidity, patients with full working capacity, and an excellent medium-term prognosis [8]. Despite the importance of these studies, their data should not be extrapolated to patients who currently live in large urban centers.

The rate of disease progression from ICF to CHD is poorly known. The few prospective studies that addressed this issue considerably differed in the study population age, number of cases, length of follow-up, geographical area, living in endemic area with or without active vectorial transmission, and migration to urban areas. More recent studies using methods similar to those of the present study were conducted in different countries (Brazil, Argentina, and Venezuela) with different geographic, climatic, and ecosystem configurations and with different vector transmission dynamics, which may explain the differences in the reported rates of disease progression [9–22].

Thus, the objective of this study was to estimate the rate of progression from the ICF to CHD in a large Brazilian urban cohort of chronic CD patients and to identify the factors that are associated with CD progression.

2. Methods

This is a retrospective observational study of a historical cohort, consisting of patients diagnosed with the ICF of CD, followed at the outpatient center of the Evandro Chagas National Institute of Infectious Diseases (Instituto Nacional de Infectologia Evandro Chagas—INI) of the Oswaldo Cruz Foundation (Fundação Oswaldo Cruz—Fiocruz), from November 1986 to December 2007 and followed until December 2008. Patients who were not followed for at least one year or without a paired electrocardiogram (ECG) during the follow-up were excluded from the study. The study was approved by the INI/Fiocruz Research Ethics Committee (054/2011).

Serological diagnosis of CD was confirmed when two serological techniques were reactive: Indirect immunofluorescence (titer >1/40) and enzyme-linked immunosorbent assay (reactivity index >1.2). All patients with a confirmed diagnosis were subjected to an initial evaluation protocol, which included: Epidemiological history, directed anamnesis, physical examination focused on CD-related cardiovascular signs and symptoms, 12-lead ECG, and two-dimensional echocardiogram with Doppler (ECHO).

Some patients were submitted to parasitological evaluation through xenodiagnosis (xeno) as recommended by Cerisola et al. [23]. ECG was performed on admission to the cohort and repeated annually in all patients. The Minnesota Code Manual of Electrocardiographic Findings [24], modified for CD, was used to standardize the ECG interpretation. The electrocardiogram changes considered compatible with Chagas disease followed the criteria recommended by the 2nd Brazilian Consensus on Chagas Disease, 2015: 2nd- and 3rd-degree right bundle-branch block, associated or not to left anterior fascicular block; frequent ventricular premature beats; polymorphous or repetitive nonsustained ventricular tachycardia; 2nd- and 3rd-degree atrioventricular block; sinus bradycardia with heart rate 50 bpm; sinus node dysfunction; 2nd- and 3rd-degree left bundle-branch block; atrial fibrillation; electrical inactive area; or primary ST-T wave changes [25]. The echocardiographic examination included parasternal and cross-sectional views and 2-, 4-, and 3- chamber apical views and variations to identify wall motion abnormalities. Left ventricular global systolic function was assessed by the Simpson method and classified as normal, mild, moderate, or severely depressed [26]. Patients' follow-up included at least one annual medical visit and one annual ECG.

3. Data Analysis

Categorical variables were described as the frequency (percentage) and numerical variables as the mean and standard deviation. The Chi-squared test was used to compare categorical variables. Cumulative incidence, which is expressed as the proportion between those who were exposed at baseline and those who presented the studied end-point during the observation period, and incidence density, which is expressed as the number of events during the time of exposure of each individual, were described in the incidence analysis. Uni and multivariate Cox analyses were performed to identify CD progression predictors. Kaplan–Meier survival curves stratified according to the presence or absence of variables associated with CD progression were constructed and compared using the log-rank test. The program IBM®SPSS®Statistics 21 (New York, NY, USA) was used, setting the significance level at 5% for all tests.

4. Results

Of a total of 1606 patients with CD, followed at INI/Fiocruz, from November 1986 to December 2008, 701 met the inclusion criteria. Of these patients, 151 were excluded because they were not followed for at least 1 year or because they did not perform a second ECG during the follow-up period. The final studied population consisted of 550 patients (44.2 ± 11.5 years, 48.9% men) who were followed for a mean period of 65 ± 42 months.

Most patients were born in the Bahia (BA) and Minas Gerais (MG) states, accounting for 23.3% and 22.9% of the subjects, respectively. Most patients had been away from an endemic area for more than 20 years (54.4%). At baseline, 519 (94.4%) patients had a normal ECHO. Xeno tests were performed in 107 patients, of whom 34.6% were positive. Of the 550 patients followed, 99 (18%) were treated with benznidazole at baseline.

A total of 37 patients progressed to CHD according to new ECG changes, resulting in a 6.7% cumulative incidence and 1.48 by 100 patients/year incidence density. The mean age at CHD progression was 56.2 years. Patients who progressed to CHD were older, had a longer mean follow-up time, a higher prevalence of associated heart disease, were more likely born in the Bahia and Minas Gerais states, had lived more than 20 years away from endemic areas, and showed positive xeno compared to non-progressors (Table 1).

Table 1. Baseline characteristics of progressor and non-progressor patients. Age and follow-up time are expressed as mean ± standard deviation; ¥ n = 107 (7 progressors and 100 non-progressors); BA: Bahia State: MG: Minas Gerais State.

Variable	Total Patients (n = 550)	Progressors (n = 37)	Non-Progressors (n = 512)	p-Value
Age (years)	44.25 ± 11.55	47.8 ± 12.2	44 ± 11.5	0.05
Follow-up time (months)	65 ± 42	73 ± 48	64 ± 42	0.25
Male	269 (48.9%)	18 (48.7%)	251 (48.9%)	0.97
Hypertension	180 (32.7%)	16 (43.2%)	164 (32%)	0.16
Diabetes	23 (4.2%)	4 (10.8%)	19 (3.7%)	0.06
Dyslipidemia	133 (24.2%)	13 (35.1%)	120 (23.4%)	0.11
Associated heart disease	16 (2.9%)	6 (16.2%)	10 (1.95%)	<0.001
From State of BA/MG	254 (46.2%)	24 (64.9%)	230 (44.8%)	0.018
Living in a non-endemic area ≥20 anos	299 (54.4%)	29 (78.4%)	270 (52.6%)	0.002
Positive xenodiagnosis ¥	37 (34.6%)	6/7 (85.7%)	31/100 (31%)	0.007
Previous benzonidazol treatment	99 (18%)	6 (16.2%)	93 (18.1%)	0.77
Altered echocardiogram	31 (5.6%)	3 (8.1%)	28 (5.5%)	0.46

Among the 37 progressors, 26 (70%) presented comorbidities: 16 patients had systemic arterial hypertension (SAH), including 6 with left ventricular hypertrophy (LVH) on ECHO; 12 patients had dyslipidemia; and 4 patients presented diabetes mellitus (DM). Fifteen patients presented only one comorbidity, 6 presented with 2 comorbidities, and 5 presented with 3 comorbidities. Four cardiovascular events occurred in these patients: Acute myocardial infarction (AMI), total atrioventricular block (TAVB), atrial fibrillation (AF), and heart failure (HF). One death was associated with ischemic heart disease.

Among the new changes diagnosed on follow-up ECGs, 67.5% were intraventricular conduction disorders (IVCD), followed by primary ST-T wave changes (32.4%). and ventricular arrhythmias (29.7%) (Table 2). In total, 30% of patients had an abnormal ECHO at baseline, and LV wall motion abnormalities and LVH were the predominant findings. There were no significant differences in alterations on ECHO between progressors and non-progressors at baseline. Among the 37 progressors, 7 were subjected to xeno, including 6 positive and 1 negative, and 6 received specific treatment with benznidazole at the beginning of their follow-up.

The five variables that initially showed differences between progressors and non-progressors at baseline were tested by univariate Cox regression, remaining associated with progression to CHD, age, associated heart disease, and living more than 20 years away from endemic areas. After the multivariate Cox regression model, including these three variables, only associated heart disease remained independently associated with progression to CHD (Table 3). Figure 1 shows the Kaplan–Meier curve stratified according to the presence of associated heart disease (log-rank test $p < 0.001$).

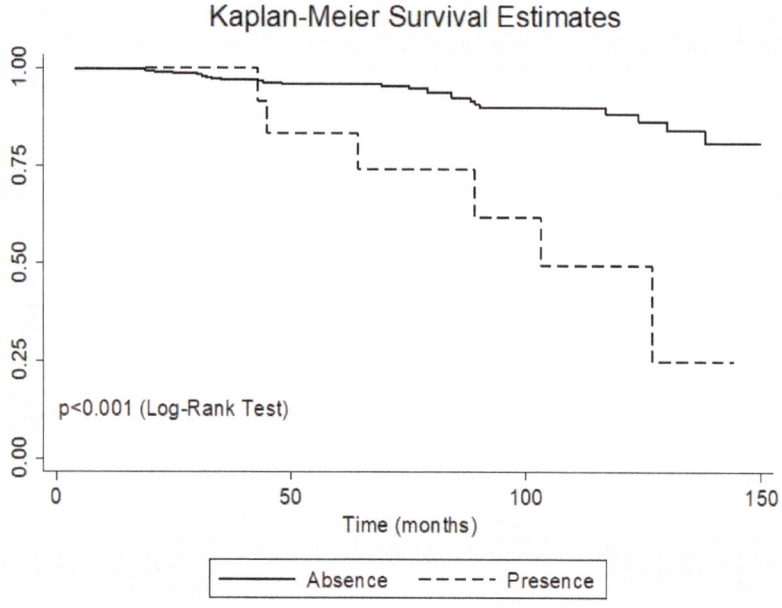

Figure 1. Kaplan–Meier survival curve stratified by the presence of non-chagasic cardiomyopathy.

Table 2. Age, sex, follow-up time, and electrocardiogram (ECG) and echocardiogram (ECHO) abnormalities among those patients that progressed to the cardiac form (n = 37) AF: atrial fibrillation; AFL: atrial flutter; AS: sinus arrhythmia; AVB1°: first degree atrioventricular block; EIA: electrical inactive area; FPAC = frequent premature atrial complex; FVPB: frequent ventricular premature beats; IPAC-isolated premature atrial complex; IVPB: isolated ventricular premature beats; LAFB: left anterior fascicular block; LBBB1°: first-degree left bundle-branch block; LBBB2°: second-degree left bundle-branch block; LBBB3°: third degree left bundle-branch block; LV: QRS low voltage; MAP: migratory atrial pacemaker; PRA: primary ST-T wave changes; RBBB1°: first-degree right bundle-branch block; RBBB3°: third-degree right bundle-branch block; SBRAD: sinus bradycardia with heart rate 50 bpm; SRA: secondary ST-T wave changes; ANEU: aneurism; DIS: dysfunction; LVH: left ventricular hypertrophy; LVEF: left ventricular ejection fraction; SEG DIS: segmental dysfunction.

ID	Sex	Time to Progression (Months)	Age at Beginning (Years)	Age at Progression (Years)	Initial ECG	ECG at Progression	Initial ECHO	Initial ECHO Abnormality	Initial LVEF	ECHO at Progression
1	M	48	67	69	NORMAL	PRA	NORMAL	-	77%	NORMAL
2	M	127	45	55	NORMAL	RBBB3° + LAFB + IVPB	ABNORMAL	LVH	56%	ANEU + LVEF = 52%
3	M	75	33	39	NORMAL	PRA + RBBB2°	NORMAL	-	63%	NORMAL
4	M	84	35	42	NORMAL	RBBB3° + FVPB	NORMAL	-	71%	LVH
5	M	22	56	58	MAP	FVPB	ABNORMAL	SEG DIS	50%	NORMAL
6	M	43	43	45	NORMAL	RBBB2°	NORMAL	-	67%	NORMAL
7	M	35	47	50	SBRAD + AVB1°	PRA + FVPB	ABNORMAL	SEG DIS	55%	LVH + DIS/LVEF = 40%
8	F	90	74	81	AVB1°	LAFB + AFL	ABNORMAL	SEG DIS	54%	NORMAL
9	M	89	59	66	NORMAL	AF	NORMAL	-	64%	LVH + DIS/LVEF = 53%
10	M	178	44	59	NORMAL	PRA + AVB1° + LAFB + LBBB2°	NORMAL	-	64%	DIS/LVEF = 54%
11	M	117	20	29	AS	LBBB3°	ABNORMAL	LVH	56%	LVH + DIS/LVEF = 49%
12	F	25	37	39	SRA	EIA	ABNORMAL	ANEU	61%	NORMAL
13	F	43	57	60	SBRAD + SRA	PRA	ABNORMAL	LVH	74%	NORMAL
14	M	31	29	31	LAFB	PRA + LAFB	NORMAL	-	70%	NORMAL
15	M	79	20	26	NORMAL	SBRAD + AVB1° + RBBB3° + LAFB	NORMAL	-	69%	NORMAL
16	F	103	56	63	IVPB	PRA + IPAC	NORMAL	-	84%	NORMAL
17	F	84	42	49	IVPB	RBBB3°	ABNORMAL	LVH	73%	NORMAL
18	F	88	54	61	AVB1°	LBBB2°	NORMAL	-	79%	LVH
19	F	44	47	51	RBBB1°	PRA +LBBB1° + LV	NORMAL	-	72%	NORMAL
20	M	138	55	66	NORMAL	AF	NORMAL	-	63%	ANEU
21	F	89	60	70	LBBB1°	RBBB2° + LAFB + IVPB	ABNORMAL	LVH	75%	NORMAL
22	M	33	60	63	NORMAL	EIA	NORMAL	-	69%	NORMAL
23	M	168	50	54	NORMAL	RBBB2° + LAFB	NORMAL	-	73%	NORMAL
24	F	124	40	50	NORMAL	PRA + FVPB	NORMAL	-	68%	LVH + DIS/LVEF = 54%
25	F	19	48	50	SBRAD + IPAC	SBRAD + RBBB2°	NORMAL	-	66%	NORMAL
26	F	21	43	45	LAFB + LV	RBBB2° + LAFB + LV	NORMAL	-	74%	NORMAL
27	F	19	43	45	NORMAL	RBBB2° + LAFB	NORMAL	-	64%	LVH

Table 2. Cont.

ID	Sex	Time to Progression (Months)	Age at Beginning (Years)	Age at Progression (Years)	Initial ECG	ECG at Progression	Initial ECHO	Initial ECHO Abnormality	Initial LVEF	ECHO at Progression
28	F	192	50	66	NORMAL	PRA + SBRAD	NORMAL	-	68%	NORMAL
29	F	30	31	34	SBRAD + LBBBI°	PRA + LAFB + FVPB	NORMAL	-	65%	NORMAL
30	F	4	64	64	SRA	LBBB3°	NORMAL	-	60%	NORMAL
31	M	45	57	61	AS	MAP + LBBBI° + IPAC + FVPB	ABNORMAL	LVH	74%	DIS/LVEF = 52%
32	M	32	37	39	SBRAD	LBBB3° + MAP	NORMAL	-	63%	NORMAL
33	M	64	60	65	SRA	RBBB3° + LAFB + FVPB	ABNORMAL	LVH	58%	NORMAL
34	F	31	50	52	NORMAL	PRA	ABNORMAL	LVH	74%	NORMAL
35	F	79	54	60	NORMAL	RBBB2°	NORMAL	-	62%	NORMAL
36	F	69	52	57	NORMAL	RBBB2° + FVPB	NORMAL	-	65%	NORMAL
37	F	130	50	55	NORMAL	RBBB3° + LAFB + FVPB	NORMAL	-	64%	NORMAL

Table 3. Univariate and multivariate Cox regression model for progression from the indeterminate to cardiac form.

Variable	Univariate Analysis		Multivariate Analysis	
	HR (95% CI)	p-Value	HR (95% CI)	p-Value
Age	1.03 (1.00 to 1.06)	0.03	1.02 (0.98 to 1.05)	0.37
Associated heart disease	5.37 (2.22 to 13.00)	<0.001	4.10 (1.65 to 10.20)	0.002
From State of BA/MG	1.68 (0.85 to 3.34)	0.14	–	–
Living in a non-endemic area ≥20 years	2.44 (1.10 to 5.38)	0.03	1.81 (0.77 to 4.26)	0.18
Positive xenodiagnosis	1.07 (0.35 to 3.29)	0.89	–	–

5. Discussion

Our study described a lower CD progression rate than previous studies. Among the reasons that can ascertain this difference are the different ECG criteria used to define CHD, reinfection in endemic areas, mean age at baseline, and follow-up time.

The changes in ECG considered as ECG progression criteria described in most previous studies included changes, such as secondary ST-T wave changes, first-degree atrioventricular and intraventricular conduction disorders, and isolated supraventricular and ventricular extra systoles, which are no longer considered diagnostic of CHD, as described in the guidelines followed in the present study. This fact may have contributed to an overestimation of CD progression in these studies.

Reinfection could influence CD progression to CHD among patients included in field studies conducted in the 1960s and 1970s, when CD control measures were still not effective [11].

The mean age of patients at baseline may also influence the difference in results between studies. Patients of a younger age have more time to present CD progression during their follow-up [27,28]. The mean age of the patients followed in our study was 44.2 years, while in field studies performed in the 1960s and 1970s, the mean age was younger than 25 years, including children and adolescents, thereby accounting for a higher number of progressions. In turn, from the 1990s, studies have tended to include adults ≥40 years and elderly people, who likely had already progressed to chronic CHD, thus accounting for the lower rate of progression found in our cohort.

The follow-up observation time is also a key variable, which accounts for differences in the rates of progression to CHD found between studies considering the natural history of CD. A retrospective cohort study of healthy blood donors showed that the rate of progression to CHD was 1.85% per year, defining that a 10-year follow-up period would be sufficient to identify the incidence of CHD [29]. The follow-up time of published studies ranges from 3 to 13 years, while the follow-up time of our study was 22 years, which is the longest follow-up time of longitudinal studies thus far. Even our reported loss to follow-up of 22% did not decrease the value of our long-term follow-up, as 78% of our patients had a follow-up of at least 10 years.

Women slightly prevailed (51.1%) in our sample, as in other studies [11,13,18,20,21]. Male sex was associated with progression to CHD in a previous field study [30], which was not confirmed in our study.

Most patients of our cohort were long-term residents of the metropolitan region of the state of Rio de Janeiro, similar to those described in other urban cohorts [19,21,22]. However, they were mostly migrants from 19 endemic Brazilian states, mainly Bahia and Minas Gerais. These states present the highest prevalence of CD and CHD [31], which may be the result of the varying pathogenic degrees of *T. cruzi* [15]. Regional differences are associated with both disease severity and the predominance of clinical forms due to factors linked to the parasitized individual (immune status, nutritional status, genetic factors, and physical effort) and to other factors related to the parasite (different strains of *T. cruzi*, parasitism intensity, and reinfections) [32,33].

Considering the role that circulating *T. cruzi* can play in the evolution of CHD, we assessed the relationship between positive xeno and ECG progression. The frequency of positive xeno in our study was similar to that of previous studies with chronic patients [34]. Nevertheless, no association was found between positive parasitemia and ECG progression, most likely due to the limited number of patients subjected to this evaluation protocol. The absence of an association between parasitemia and chronic CD progression was also described in other longitudinal studies [35].

Regarding comorbidities, the percentage of SAH, DM, and dyslipidemia in this cohort is similar to the estimated prevalence of these comorbidities in the Brazilian population, and, as described in other series of patients with CD, none of them were associated with ECG progression [36,37]. Some studies demonstrated no risk in the coexistence of SAH and CD [38]. In our cohort, 16 patients (2.9%) had associated heart disease at baseline, most often LVH, with minimal or no degree of LV systolic dysfunction. We identified five cases of ischemic heart disease with three occurrences of acute myocardial infarction (AMI). The electrocardiographic changes eventually associated with these events (electrically inactive zones or isolated primary repolarization changes) were not considered criteria for CD progression but manifestations of the associated heart disease. Although the number of patients with associated heart disease at baseline was low, those patients had an increased risk of progression to CHD diagnosed by ECG changes typical of CD, and associated heart disease was the only independent risk factor for progression to CHD.

The most frequent ECG change found in those who progressed to CHD in our study was IVCD, followed by primary ST-T wave changes, and ventricular arrhythmias. This finding corroborates several studies in which the same ECG changes were the most frequently found in CHD [39,40]. Regarding progression to CHD, other studies described primary ST-T wave changes and ICD as the most frequent findings [9,21].

Regarding ECHO, segmental changes predominated in those who had an altered ECHO at baseline, whereas diffuse changes predominated in patients who had a normal ECHO at baseline. This suggests that echocardiographic alterations indicative of an incipient process of impaired global systolic function may be the physiopathogenic basis of the electrocardiographic changes identified among progressors. In a previous study of the same cohort, the prevalence of LV aneurysm was 24% among patients with an abnormal electrocardiogram and 2% among patients with a normal ECG [41]. In addition, diastolic functioning has been described as being altered in up to 10% of patients with a normal ECG in our institution [42].

Despite the progression to CHD by ECG changes, none of the 37 patients who started the follow-up with ICF and progressed to CHD showed symptoms or signs compatible with CD. The clinical cardiological events (AMI, AF, TAVB, and HF) that affected progressors were apparently more related to associated heart diseases and/or to aging. The only case of HF was related to tachycardiomyopathy associated with AF in an elderly patient with severe SAH. AF and TAVB also occurred in two elderly patients (66 and 85 years, respectively). The only death was recorded in a patient who had an AMI, which corroborates the good prognosis of patients with ICF described in longitudinal studies in which mortality rates are similar to that of individuals of the same age group without CD [43]. Regarding age, ECG changes that occur in the general population in primary care are associated with age and comorbidities [44]. Therefore, we should consider that in CD cohorts with elderly patients, the onset of new cardiovascular events could be expected due to the ageing process, including degenerative changes in the conduction system, or complications from other morbidities, such as SAH and atherosclerotic disease. In fact, age was associated with CD progression after univariate analysis. However, comorbidities are also highly prevalent among elderly individuals, and after multivariate analysis, age was no longer associated with CD progression.

The increase in life expectancy observed in individuals infected with *T. cruzi* and the migration of most of the population from rural areas to large urban centers exposes these individuals to several lifestyle habits that favor the development of chronic degenerative changes, such as obesity, insulin resistance, arterial hypertension, and dyslipidemia, which, in combination with nutritional aspects and aging, significantly increase the risk of cardiovascular events and death [45,46]. Over the past few decades, studies have increasingly shown that patients with CD have comorbidities that become increasingly more frequent as this population ages [5]. The difficulty in implementing healthy habits makes them more vulnerable to the concomitant onset of other chronic diseases [47]. Another key issue is that the higher the number of comorbidities is, the greater the adverse impact on prognosis will be with the increase in morbidity and mortality. Ischemic heart disease worsens ventricular function and can exacerbate the clinical symptoms of CD, worsening the prognosis. Importantly, coronary artery disease increases the risk of sudden death, which is already high in CHD. As in the general population, SAH is the most prevalent comorbidity, and these hypertensive patients are 40% more likely to present with HF than non-hypertensive patients [36,48].

The findings of the present study indicate that the rate of ICF progression to CHD is low and lower than the rates described in previous studies conducted in endemic and rural areas, albeit compatible with studies conducted from the 2000s, in urban and non-endemic areas. The presence of associated heart disease, especially LVH, was independently associated with ECG progression.

However, our study is limited by the characteristic slow progression of patients with CD and ICF, which resulted in a low number of events during the follow-up. The low number of events makes the identification of other potential variables associated with ECG progression difficult. Thus, further studies with a longer follow-up period or larger number of patients are necessary to better identify the variables associated with progression.

Author Contributions: Conceptualization: A.M.H.-M., S.S.X. and A.S.d.S. Provided clinical date—A.M.H.-M., S.S.X. and A.S.d.S. Formal analyses—G.M.S.d.S., M.F.F.M. and A.S.d.S. Management the patient—A.M.H.-M., S.S.X., R.M.S., L.H.C.S., M.T.d.H., H.H.V., A.R.d.C., F.d.S.N.S.M., P.E.A.A.d.B., A.S.d.S. Writing—A.M.H-M. and A.S.d.S., Writing—Revision—R.M.S. All authors have read and agreed to the published version of the manuscript.

Funding: This research received no external funding.

Conflicts of Interest: The authors declare no conflict of interest.

References

1. Pan American Health Organization. PAHO Issues New Guide for Diagnosis and Treatment of Chagas Disease. 7 January 2019. Available online: https://www.paho.org/hq/index.php?option=com_content&view=article&id=14906:paho-issues-new-guide-for-diagnosis-and-treatment-of-chagas-disease&Itemid=135&lang=pt (accessed on 2 March 2020). (In Spanish)
2. Gascon, J.; Bern, C.; Pinazo, M.-J. Chagas disease in Spain, the United States and other non-endemic countries. *Acta Trop.* **2010**, *115*, 22–27.
3. Cavalcante dos Santos, V.R.; de Meis, J.; Savino, W.; Azevedo Andrade, J.A.; dos Santos Vieira, J.R.; Coura, J.R.; Verissimo Junqueira, A.C. Acute Chagas disease in the state of Pará, Amazon Region: Is it increasing? *Mem. Inst. Oswaldo Cruz* **2018**, *113*, 1–6.
4. Francisco-González, L.; Rubio-San-Simón, A.; González-Tomé, M.I.; Manzanares, Á.; Epalza, C.; del Mar Santos, M.; Gastañaga, T.; Merino, P.; Ramos-Amador, J.T. Congenital transmission of Chagas disease in a non-endemic area, is an early diagnosis possible? *PLoS ONE* **2019**, *14*, 1–7. [CrossRef] [PubMed]
5. Vizzoni, A.G.; Varela, M.C.; Sangenis, L.H.C.; Hasslocher-Moreno, A.M.; do Brasil, P.E.A.A.; Saraiva, R.M. Ageing with Chagas disease: An overview of an urban Brazilian cohort in Rio de Janeiro. *Parasit Vectors* **2018**, *11*, 2–8. [CrossRef] [PubMed]
6. Martins-Melo, F.R.; Ramos, A.N.; Alencar, C.H.; Heukelbach, J. Prevalence of Chagas disease in Brazil: A systematic review and meta-analysis. *Acta Trop.* **2014**, *130*, 167–174.
7. Biolo, A.; Ribeiro, A.L.; Clausell, N. Chagas cardiomyopathy—Where do we stand after a hundred years? *Prog. Cardiovasc. Dis.* **2010**, *52*, 300–316. [CrossRef]
8. Ribeiro, A.L.P.; da Costa Rocha, M.O. Indeterminate form of Chagas' disease: Considerations about diagnosis and prognosis. *Rev. Soc. Bras. Med. Trop.* **1998**, *31*, 301–314. [CrossRef]
9. Puigbó, J.J.; Nava Rhode, J.R.; Garcia Barrios, H.; Gil Yepez, C. Cuatro años de estudio longitudinal de una comunidad rural con endemicidad chagasica. *Bol. Oficina Sanit. Panam.* **1968**, *66*, 112–120.
10. Moleiro, F.; Pifano, F.; Anselmi, A.; Ruesta, V. La dinamica epidemiologica de la enfermedad de Chagas en el valle de los Naranjos. Estado Carabobo, Venezuela. *Arch. Venezoelanos Med. Trop. Parasitol. Medica* **1973**, *5*, 47–83.

11. Macedo, V. Influência da exposição à reinfecção na evolução da doença de Chagas. Estudo longitudinal de 5 anos. *Rev. Patol. Trop.* **1976**, *5*, 33–116.
12. Pereira, J.B.; Willcox, H.P.; Coura, J.R. Morbidity of Chagas disease: III. Six-year longitudinal study, at Virgem da Lapa, MG, Brazil. *Mem. Inst. Oswaldo Cruz* **1985**, *80*, 63–71. [CrossRef] [PubMed]
13. Coura, J.R.; de Abreu, L.L.; Pereira, J.B.; Willcox, H.P. Morbidity in Chagas' disease: IV. Longitudinal study of 10 years in Pains and Iguatama, Minas Gerais, Brazil. *Mem. Inst. Oswaldo Cruz* **1985**, *80*, 73–80. [CrossRef] [PubMed]
14. Espinosa, R.; Carrasco, H.A.; Belandria, F.; Fuenmayor, A.M.; Molina, C.; González, R.; Martínez, O. Life expectancy analysis in patients with Chagas' disease: Prognosis after one decade (1973–1983). *Int. J. Cardiol.* **1985**, *8*, 45–56. [CrossRef]
15. Pereira, J.B.; da Cunha, R.V.; Willcox, H.P.F.; Coura, J.R. Evolução da cardiopatia chagásica crônica humana no sertão do Estado da Paraíba, Brasil, no período de 4, 5 anos. *Rev. Soc. Bras. Med. Trop.* **1990**, *23*, 141–147. [CrossRef]
16. Mota, E.A.; Guimarães, A.C.; Santana, O.O.; Sherlock, I.; Hoff, R.; Weller, T.H. A nine year prospective study of Chagas' disease in a defined rural population in northeast Brazil. *Am. J. Trop. Med. Hyg.* **1990**, *42*, 429–440. [CrossRef]
17. Madoery, R.J.; Dománico, A.; Marcelino, A.; Madoery, C. Alteraciones electrocardiográficas durante el período intermedio, latente o indeterminado de la enfermedad de Chagas: Consideraciones evolutivas. *Rev Lat Cardiol* **1992**, *13*, 55–59.
18. Viotti, R.; Vigliano, C.; Armenti, H.; Segura, E. Treatment of chronic Chagas' disease with benznidazole: Clinical and serologic evolution of patients with long-term follow-up. *Am. Heart J.* **1994**, *127*, 151–162. [CrossRef]
19. Da Silva, M.A.D.; Costa, J.M.; Barbosa, J.M.; Cabral, F.; Fragata Filho, A.A.; Correa, E.B.; Borges Filho, R.; Sousa, J.E.M. Fase crônica da doença de Chagas: Aspectos clínicos e evolutivos. *Arq. Bras. Cardiol.* **1994**, *63*, 281–285.
20. Castro, C.; Prata, A.; Macedo, V. A folow-up period of 13 years prospective study in 190 chagasic patients of Mambaí, Goiás, State, Brazil. *Rev. Soc. Bras. Med. Trop.* **2001**, *34*, 309–318. [CrossRef]
21. Ianni, B.M.; Arteaga, E.; Frimm, C.D.C.; Barretto, A.C.P.; Mady, C. Chagas' heart disease: Evolutive evaluation of electrocardiographic and echocardiographic parameters in patients with the indeterminate form. *Arq. Bras. Cardiol.* **2001**, *77*, 59–62. [CrossRef]
22. Viotti, R.; Vigliano, C.; Lococo, B.; Bertocchi, G.; Petti, M.; Alvarez, M.G.; Postan, M.; Armenti, A. Long-term cardiac outcomes of treating chronic Chagas disease with benznidazole versus no treatment: A nonrandomized trial. *Ann. Intern. Med.* **2006**, *144*, 724–734. [CrossRef] [PubMed]
23. Cerisola, J.A.; Rohwedder, R.W.; Del Prado, C.E. Yield of xenodiagnosis in human chronic Chagas' infection using nymphs of different species of triatomid bugs. *Bol. Chil. Parasitol.* **1971**, *26*, 57. [PubMed]
24. Prineas, R.J.; Crow, R.S.; Blackburn, H. *The Minnesota Manual of Electrographic Findings*; John Wright: Bristol, UK, 1982; Available online: https://books.google.com.hk/books?id=8s8Gfynp7AsC&pg=PA46&lpg=PA46&dq=The+Minnesota+manual+of+electrographic+findings.+Bristol:+John+Wright&source=bl&ots=_xfZPrRqMg&sig=ACfU3U2gsjEQE6btQ8uIuJbAh9BT_8wmBA&hl=zhCN&sa=X&redir_esc=y&sourceid=cndr#v=onepage&q=The%20Minnesota%20manual%20of%20electrographic%20findings.%20Bristol%3A%20John%20Wright&f=false (accessed on 12 May 2020).
25. Dias, J.C.P.; Ramos, A.N., Jr.; Gontijo, E.D.; Luquetti, A.; Shikanai-Yasuda, M.A.; Coura, J.R.; Torres, R.M.; da Cunha Melo, J.R.; de Almeida, E.A.; Correia Filho, D.; et al. 2nd Brazilian Consensus on Chagas Disease, 2015. *Epidemiol. Serv. Saúde* **2016**, *25*, 7–86. [PubMed]
26. Cerqueira, M.; Weissman, N.; Dilsizian, V.; Jacobs, A.; Kaul, S.; Laskey, W.; Pennell, D.; Rumberger, J.; Ryan, T.; Verani, M. Standardized Myocardial Segmentation and Nomenclature for Tomographic Imaging of the Heart. A Statement for Healthcare Professionals From the Cardiac Imaging Committee of the Council on Clinical Cardiology of the American Heart Association. *Circulation* **2002**, *105*, 539–542.
27. Dias, J.C.P. História natural da doença de Chagas. *Arq. Bras. Cardiol.* **1995**, *65*, 359–366.
28. Dias, E.; Laranja, F.S.; Nobrega, G. Doença de Chagas. *Mem. Inst. Oswaldo Cruz* **1945**, *43*, 495–581. [CrossRef]
29. Sabino, E.C.; Ribeiro, A.L.; Salemi, V.M.; Oliveira, C.D.L.; Antunes, A.P.; Menezes, M.M.; Ianni, B.M.; Nastari, L.; Fernandes, F.; Patavino, G.M.; et al. Ten-year Incidence of Chagas cardiomyopathy among asymptomatic, T. cruzi seropositive former blood donors. *Circulation* **2013**, *127*, 1105–1115. [CrossRef]

30. Pereira, J.B.; Wilcox, H.P.F.; Coura, J.R. Evolução da cardiopatia chagásica crônica. Influência da parasitemia. *Rev. Soc. Bras. Med. Trop.* **1992**, *25*, 101–108. [CrossRef]
31. Dias, J.C.P.; Machado, E.M.M.; Fernandes, A.L.; Vinhaes, M.C. General situation and perspectives of Chagas disease in Northeastern Region, Brazil. *Cad. Saúde Pública* **2000**, *16*, 13–34. [CrossRef]
32. Bellini, M.F.; Silistino-Souza, R.; Varella-Garcia, M.; de Azeredo-Oliveira, M.T.V.; Silva, A.E. Biologic and genetics aspects of Chagas disease at endemic areas. *J. Trop. Med.* **2012**, *2012*, 1–11. [CrossRef]
33. Ayo, C.M.; de Oliveira Dalalio, M.M.; Visentainer, J.E.L.; Reis, P.G.; Sippert, E.Â.; Jarduli, L.R.; Alves, H.V.; Sell, A.M. Genetic susceptibility to Chagas disease: An overview about the infection and about the association between disease and the immune response genes. *BioMed Res. Int.* **2013**, *2013*, 1–13. [CrossRef] [PubMed]
34. Portela-Lindoso, A.; Shikanai-Yasuda, M. Chronic Chagas' disease: From xenodiagnosis and hemoculture to polymerase chain reaction. *Rev. Saúde Pública* **2003**, *37*, 107–115. [CrossRef] [PubMed]
35. De Castro, C.N.; Prata, A.; Macedo, V. Influência da parasitemia na evolução da doença de Chagas crônica. *Rev. Soc. Bras. Med. Trop.* **2005**, *38*, 01–06. [CrossRef] [PubMed]
36. Gurgel, C.; Miguel Junior, A.; Mendes, C.R.; Zerbini, C.O.; Carcioni, T.M. Frequency of arterial hypertension in chronic Chagas' disease. A retrospective study. *Arq. Bras. Cardiol.* **2003**, *81*, 541–544. [CrossRef]
37. Guariento, M.E.; Ramos, C.M.; Gontijo, J.A.; Carvalhal, S.S. Chagas disease and primary arterial hypertension. *Arq. Bras. Cardiol.* **1993**, *60*, 71–75.
38. Ianni, B.M.; Mady, C.; Arteaga, E.; Fernandes, F. Cardiovascular Diseases Observed During Follow-up of a Group of Patients in Undetermined Form of Chagas' Disease. *Arq. Bras. Cardiol.* **1998**, *71*, 21–24. [CrossRef]
39. Marcolino, M.S.; Palhares, D.M.; Ferreira, L.R.; Ribeiro, A.L. Electrocardiogram and Chagas Disease. A Large Population Database of Primary Care Patients. *Glob. HEART* **2015**, *10*, 167–172. [CrossRef]
40. Brito, B.O.F.; Ribeiro, A.L.P. Electrocardiogram in Chagas disease. *Rev. Soc. Bras. Med. Trop.* **2018**, *51*, 570–577. [CrossRef]
41. Xavier, S.S.; de Sousa, A.S.; do Brasil, P.E.A.A.; Gabriel, F.G.; de Holanda, M.T.; Hasslocher-Moreno, A. Apical Aneurysm in the Chronic Phase of Chagas Disease: Prevalence and Prognostic Value in an Urban Cohort of 1053 Patients. *Rev. SOCERJ* **2005**, *18*, 351–356.
42. Nascimento, C.; Gomes, V.; Silva, S.; Santos, C.; Chambela, M.; Madeira, F.; Holanda, M.; Brasil, P.; Sousa, A.; Xavier, S.; et al. Left atrial and left ventricular diastolic function in chronic Chagas disease. *J. Am. Soc. Echocardiogr.* **2013**, *26*, 1424–1433. [CrossRef]
43. Maguire, J.H.; Hoff, R.; Sherlock, I.; Guimaraes, A.C.; Sleigh, A.C.; Ramos, N.B.; Mott, K.E.; Weller, T.H. Cardiac morbidity and mortality due to Chagas' disease: Prospective electrocardiographic study of a Brazilian community. *Circulation* **1987**, *75*, 1140–1145. [CrossRef] [PubMed]
44. Marcolino, M.S.; Palhares, D.M.F.; Alkmim, M.B.M.; Ribeiro, A.L. Prevalence of normal electrocardiograms in primary care patients. *Rev. Assoc. Médica Bras.* **2014**, *60*, 236–241. [CrossRef] [PubMed]
45. Santos, J.P.; Lima-Costa, M.F.; Peixoto, S.V. Nutritional aspects associated with chronic Trypanosoma cruzi (Chagas 1909) infection among older adults: Bambuí Project. *Cad Saúde Pública* **2013**, *29*, 1141–1148. [CrossRef] [PubMed]
46. Geraix, J.; Ardisson, L.P.; Marcondes-Machado, J.; Pereira, P.C.M. Clinical and nutritional profile of individuals with Chagas disease. *Braz. J. Infect. Dis.* **2007**, *11*, 411–414. [CrossRef] [PubMed]
47. Jackson, Y.; Castillo, S.; Hammond, P.; Besson, M.; Brawand-Bron, A.; Urzola, D.; Gaspoz, J.-M.; Chappuis, F. Metabolic, mental health, behavioural and socioeconomic characteristics of migrants with Chagas disease in a non-endemic country. *Trop. Med. Int. Health* **2012**, *17*, 595–603. [CrossRef]
48. He, J.; Ogden, L.G.; Bazzano, L.A.; Vupputuri, S.; Loria, C.; Whelton, P.K. Risk factors for congestive heart failure in US men and women: NHANES I epidemiologic follow-up study. *Arch. Intern. Med.* **2001**, *161*, 996–1002. [CrossRef]

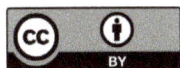

© 2020 by the authors. Licensee MDPI, Basel, Switzerland. This article is an open access article distributed under the terms and conditions of the Creative Commons Attribution (CC BY) license (http://creativecommons.org/licenses/by/4.0/).

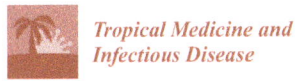

Article

Benznidazole as Prophylaxis for Chagas Disease Infection Reactivation in Heart Transplant Patients: A Case Series in Brazil

Joao Manoel Rossi Neto *, Marco Aurelio Finger and Carolina Casadei dos Santos

Instituto Dante Pazzanese de Cardiologia, Av Dante Pazzanese 500, Sao Paulo CEP 04012-909, Brazil; mfinger@uol.com.br (M.A.F.); htx@dantepazzanese.org.br (C.C.d.S.)
* Correspondence: jmrossi@sti.com.br

Received: 23 July 2020; Accepted: 12 August 2020; Published: 18 August 2020

Abstract: Background—Patients with Chagas cardiomyopathy (CC) have high mortality, and CC is a common indication for heart transplantation (HTx) in endemic countries. Chagas disease reactivation (CDR) is common after transplantation and is likely to cause adverse outcomes unless detected and treated appropriately. This study reviews our experiences with HTx among patients with CC, and the use of benznidazole (BZ) before transplantation. Methods—During the 18-year period from 1996 through 2014, 70 of 353 patients who underwent HTx (19.8%) had CC, and 53 patients met the inclusion criteria. The effectiveness of prophylactic treatment with BZ (dose of 5 mg/kg/day, two times per day, for at least four weeks and for a maximum of eight weeks) was determined based on the observed reduction in the incidence of CDR during the post-HTx period. Results—Prophylactic therapy was administered to 18/53 patients (34.0%). During the follow-up period, the incidence rate of CDR in our study was 34.0% (18/53). Based on logistic regression analysis, only prophylaxis (OR = 0.12; CI 0.02–0.76; $p = 0.025$) was considered to protect against CDR. Conclusion—Our study suggests that the use of BZ may reduce the incidence of CDR in patients undergoing HTx and warrants further investigation in a prospective, randomized trial.

Keywords: chagasic cardiomyopathy; heart transplant; chagas disease reactivation

1. Introduction

Chagas disease (CD) is a major cause of end-stage cardiomyopathy in Mexico, South America, especially in Brazil, and Central America, with 7.7 million people currently estimated to be infected in 18 countries [1]. The exodus from these rural communities in the late 20th century has resulted in a marked urbanization and globalization of CD. The number of infections in the United States and non-endemic countries in Europe and the Western Pacific Region continues to rise [2,3].

Patients with chagasic cardiomyopathy (CC) have higher mortality than patients with other etiologies of cardiomyopathy [4]; thus, CC is a common indication for heart transplantation (HTx) in endemic countries where this therapy is available.

Chagas disease reactivation (CDR) is common after HTx and is likely to cause adverse outcomes unless detected and treated appropriately [5]. In addition, acute *T. cruzi* infection causes substantial morbidity (allograft dysfunction) and mortality in the post-transplant setting if not recognized and treated early [6].

Only two drugs (benznidazole (BZ) and nifurtimox) have been shown to be effective enough to warrant widespread use in acute CD treatment [7]. Data validating the use of prophylactic therapy with BZ in patients with CD who underwent heart transplantation are lacking in the literature.

In 1995, Fragata Filho [8] suggested the necessity of elimination of the parasite with parasiticidic drugs in patients with a heart transplant and immunosuppression therapy. In addition, in 1999,

Rassi [9] described the protective effect of benznidazole (5 mg/kg/day, two times per day, 4–8 weeks) against parasite reactivation in patients chronically infected with *T. cruzi* and treated with corticoids for associated diseases. Based on these assumptions, our service began using BZ as prophylactic therapy.

This study reviews our experience with cardiac transplantation in patients with CC, emphasizing reactivation and the use of BZ before transplantation.

2. Materials and Methods

2.1. Patients and Medications

This investigation is a retrospective cohort study of heart transplant recipients with CC that was undertaken at Dante Pazzanese Institute of Cardiology and includes data compiled over a 18-year period. Between 1996 through 2014, 70 patients with CC underwent HTx. Seventeen patients were excluded because they died during hospitalization or had incomplete data. Clinical data were considered until December 2016 to guarantee at least 2 years of follow-up after transplantation.

All patients were evaluated for CD using serological screening before starting conditioning chemotherapy and transplantation.

All patients received triple drug immunosuppressive therapy that included calcineurin inhibitors (cyclosporine or tacrolimus), corticosteroids, and a third drug, which could be mycophenolate mofetil or sodium. Due to the lack of BZ that usually occurred during this period, BZ was used only when it was available and in a non-randomized way. Prophylactic therapy with BZ was prescribed at a dose of 5 mg/kg/day, two times per day, for at least 4 weeks and for a maximum of 8 weeks [9].

The protocol was approved by the review boards of the Instituto Dante Pazzanese de Cardiologia (CAAE: 47457315.8.0000.5462).

2.2. Definitions

The criteria used to diagnose CDR after HTx were evidence of parasites obtained using direct methods, such as endomyocardial biopsies (EMB), hemoculture or real-time polymerase chain reaction (PCR). None of the donors had CD.

The effectiveness of the treatment was determined based on the observed reduction in the incidence of CDR after heart transplantation.

2.3. Statistical Analysis

Continuous variables are expressed as the mean ± standard error (SE), and categorical variables are expressed as percentages. For group comparisons, the *t*-test was used for variables with a normal distribution and the Mann–Whitney test was used to compare variables without a normal distribution. For categorical variables, the χ^2 test or the Fisher exact test was applied. For the multivariate analysis, the logistic regression model was used with the Hosmer and Lemeshow test. $p < 0.05$ was considered significant. All analyses were performed using GNU PSPP (Version 0.8.5-g2d71ac) (Computer Software). Free Software Foundation. Boston, MA, USA.

3. Results

From 1996 through 2014, 353 heart transplantations were performed at Dante Pazzanese Institute of Cardiology. Seventy (19.8%) transplants were performed in patients with CC. Table 1 shows the observed differences in characteristics between the groups without prophylactic therapy (GP-) and with prophylactic therapy (GP+).

Table 1. Characteristics of patients according to benznidazole prophylactic therapy status (GP+ vs. GP−).

Variable	Total n = 53	GP− n = 35	GP+ n = 18	p-Value
Male (%)	32 (59.6)	19 (54.3)	13 (72.2)	0.261
Reactivation (%)	18 (34.0)	16 (45.7)	02 (11.1)	0.012
Corticosteroid therapy (%)	39 (75.0)	28 (80.0)	11 (61.1)	0.195
Tacrolimus therapy (%)	04 (7.5)	03 (08.6)	01 (05.6)	0.616
Cyclosporine Therapy (%)	31 (58.5)	22 (62.9)	08 (44.4)	0.252
Mycophenolate (%)	37 (69.8)	26 (74.3)	11 (61.1)	0.401
Age in years (m; SE)	48.8 (1.38)	50.4 (1.55)	46.0 (2.72)	0.141
Weight in Kg (m; SE)	62.1 (1.53)	61.6 (1.87)	62.9 (2.56)	0.671
Corticosteroid in mg (m; SE)	22.1 (2.62)	20.1 (3.30)	24.7 (4.27)	0.396
Tacrolimus in mg (m; SE)	7.0 (1.30)	7.3 (1.76)	6.0 (-)	0.742
Cyclosporine in mg (m; SE)	220.2 (11.21)	208.8 (18.06)	233.9 (11.30)	0.272
Mycophenolate in mg (m; SE)	1055.5 (59.08)	1058.7 (61.36)	1050.7 (119.55)	0.948
Ischemic time in min (m; SE)	146.2 (7.65)	152.0 (10.32)	134.8 (7.37)	0.333

m = mean; SE = standard error.

Prophylactic therapy was administered in 18 patients (34.6%). Of the 18 (34.6%) patients with CDR, the diagnosis was made using EMB (44.4%), PCR (38.9%), and hemoculture (16.7%). The main symptoms in the clinical presentation included dyspnea (33.3%), weakness (27.7%), vomiting/diarrhea (16.6%), heart failure (11.1%), and no symptoms (11.1%).

The total incidence rate of CDR in our study was 34.0% (18/53). CDR was diagnosed in 45.7% (16/35) of patients without prophylaxis and in 11.1% (02/18) of patients in the group with prophylaxis ($p = 0.012$). The mean time for CDR was 352 days (SE = 148.4).

The univariate analysis of the characteristics of patients with (CDR+) and without (CDR-) Chagas disease reactivation (Table 2) shows that both cyclosporine ($p = 0.041$) and prophylaxis ($p = 0.012$) were significant, but in the multivariate analysis, which also included variables that we thought could influence the reactivation results, only prophylaxis remained significant ($p = 0.025$) (Table 3).

Table 2. Characteristics of patients with (CDR+) and without (CDR−) Chagas disease reactivation.

Variable	CDR− n = 35	CDR+ n = 18	p-Value
Male (%)	21 (58.3)	11 (61.1)	0.938
Prophylaxis (%)	16 (45.7)	02 (11.1)	0.012
Corticosteroid therapy (%)	23 (65.7)	16 (88.9)	0.700
Tacrolimus therapy (%)	03 (08.6)	01 (05.6)	0.694
Cyclosporine Therapy (%)	17 (48.6)	14 (77.8)	0.041
Mycophenolate (%)	23 (65.7)	15 (83.3)	0.177
Age in years (m; SE)	49.3 (1.73)	47.8 (2.32)	0.626
Weight in Kg (m; SE)	61.7 (1.93)	62.9 (2.56)	0.703
Corticosteroid in mg (m; SE)	20.1 (3.30)	24.7 (4.27)	0.396
Tacrolimus in mg (m; SE)	7.3 (1.76)	6.0 (-)	0.742
Cyclosporine in mg (m; SE)	208.8 (18.06)	233.9 (11.30)	0.272
Mycophenolate in mg (m; SE)	1058.7 (61.36)	1050.7 (119.55)	0.948
Ischemic time in min (m; SE)	148.0 (10.20)	144.4 (10.94)	0.826

m = mean; SE = standard error.

Table 3. Logistic regression for CDR *.

	B	S.E.	Wald	df	Sig.	Exp(B)	Lower	Upper
Gender	−1.15	0.79	2.13	1	0.144	0.32	0.07	1.48
Prophylaxis	−2.13	0.95	5.04	1	0.025	0.12	0.02	0.76
Corticosteroid therapy	0.73	1.04	0.49	1	0.482	2.07	0.27	15.86
Tacrolimus therapy	−0.38	1.56	0.06	1	0.805	0.68	0.03	14.41
Cyclosporine therapy	1.16	0.93	1.56	1	0.212	3.19	0.52	19.69
Mycophenolate therapy	0.97	0.95	1.04	1	0.308	2.63	0.41	16.90
Constant	−0.57	1.24	0.21	1	0.648	0.57		

* Hosmer and Lemeshow test = 0.620.

4. Discussion

CDR has been described in patients with leukemia and HIV and in patients with kidney, liver, and heart transplantation. It is important to highlight that due to immunosuppression, the recipients with CD can develop CDR, and the reactivation rate of CD after HTx for CC is variable, with an incidence of 21–45% [5]. In the literature, the degree of immunosuppression was often correlated with reactivation [6,7]. At our institution, reactivation occurred in 34.6% of patients with CC. The type and dose of immunosuppression used did not differ significantly between the groups with and without CDR. Unlike the Bacal [10] study that showed that mychophenolate mofetil increased CDR in heart transplanted patients, our data failed to demonstrate which immunosuppressant could increase the chance of CDR. We hypothesized that prophylaxis might have a protective effect or that our small sample size was not powered enough to determine the effects of the immunotherapy.

Nevertheless, CDR can cause both cardiac and noncardiac (skin lesions) manifestations. The cardiac manifestations of CDR include new conduction blocks that may require pacemaker placement, valvular regurgitation, and most seriously, allograft dysfunction that can progress to cardiogenic shock and death [5,7]. In the setting of CDR after HTx, we found great clinical variability, from patients with no symptoms to patients with heart failure.

In Brazil, the most recent Clinical Protocol and Therapeutic Guidelines for Chagas Disease of the Ministry of Health [11] stated that the treatment of the acute form must be immediate. In asymptomatic cases, or when diagnostic confirmation is not possible, but with persistent suspicion, empirical treatment may be considered. The etiological treatment of the person affected with the disease in the chronic phase should be carried out in children and adolescents in the chronic indeterminate phase. For adults in the chronic indeterminate phase, the benefit of antiparasitic treatment is uncertain. In adults under 50 years old, the treatment should be considered. For Chagas heart disease in the early stages (only have changes in the electrocardiogram, with normal ejection fraction, absence of heart failure, and absence of severe arrhythmias), both treatment and untreatment with benznidazole are valid alternatives, and the decision must be shared with the patients. There is no evidence to justify the treatment of patients with advanced Chagas heart disease [11].

Prophylaxis has been demonstrated to avert transmission or reactivation in liver and renal recipients [12,13]. In patients with CC who are treated with corticoids, Rassi [9] demonstrated that for many reasons, benznidazole used as a primary chemoprophylaxis prevented increased parasitemia (evaluated by xenodiagnoses) and suggested that in immunocompromised patients with chronic CD, the use of this drug could be useful. Importantly, the myocarditis of an acute CDR patient can be easily mistaken for allograft rejection [14], and treatment with intensified immunosuppression can lead to more severe *T. cruzi* infection [7]. Unfortunately, due to a lack of raw materials or difficulty obtaining the medication for prophylactic use, BZ was unavailable for some of the study period, making it impossible to carry out a randomized study in our center.

When we started our study, PCR was not considered a consolidated diagnosis of Chagas reactivation. Since then, new scientific data have demonstrated advantages of PCR monitoring over traditional methods such as being less invasive, faster, contributing to the differential diagnosis between reactivation and rejection episodes, and preceding the clinical manifestations of reactivation by 2 or more months [15–18]. Thus, PCR is a precious tool which guides physicians to decide whether patients should begin receiving anti-parasite drugs or changes in the immunosuppression regimen. Today, the concept of reactivation must be redefined even if the patient is asymptomatic and includes an increase in parasitemia, detected either by direct parasitological techniques or by PCR [7].

To our knowledge, this study is the first reported series using BZ as prophylactic therapy before HTx in patients with CC. This study found that in the presence of prophylactic therapy, reactivation was reduced in patients with CC who were subjected to HTx (OR = 0.12, CI 0.02–0.76; p = 0.025).

Our findings reinforce the idea that monitoring for CDR should be performed routinely after HTx and during suspected reactivation episodes [7,19]. However, no scientific data are available that define exactly when such routine monitoring should be performed.

Our study has limitations common to retrospective analyses. First, the individuals enrolled in the study were not randomized to BZ therapy or placebo, and the physicians and patients were not blinded to the medical intervention. In addition, this study represents an analysis of a unique center with a small number of patients.

5. Conclusions

Our results suggest that the use of prophylactic therapy could reduce the incidence of CDR in patients who were subjected to HTx. These findings challenge the available data and warrant further randomized, double-blind studies.

Author Contributions: The authors have worked together and contributed equally to: conceptualization, methodology, formal analysis investigation, writing original draft preparation, writing—review and editing. All authors have read and agreed to the published version of the manuscript.

Funding: This research received no external funding.

Conflicts of Interest: The authors declare no conflict of interest.

References

1. Rassi, A.; Rassi, A.; Marin-Neto, J.A. Chagas disease. *Lancet* **2010**, *375*, 1388–1402. [CrossRef]
2. Bonney, K.M. Chagas disease in the 21st century: A public health success or an emerging threat? *Parasite Paris Fr.* **2014**, *21*, 11. [CrossRef] [PubMed]
3. Lidani, K.C.F.; Andrade, F.A.; Bavia, L.; Damasceno, F.S.; Beltrame, M.H.; Messias-Reason, I.J.; Sandri, T.L. Chagas disease: From discovery to a worldwide health problem. *Front. Public Health* **2019**, *7*, 166. [CrossRef] [PubMed]
4. Freitas, H.F.G.; Chizzola, P.R.; Paes, A.T.; Lima, A.C.P.; Mansur, A.J. Risk stratification in a Brazilian hospital-based cohort of 1220 outpatients with heart failure: Role of chagas' heart disease. *Int. J. Cardiol.* **2005**, *102*, 239–247. [CrossRef] [PubMed]
5. Kransdorf, E.P.; Czer, L.S.C.; Luthringer, D.J.; Patel, J.K.; Montgomery, S.P.; Velleca, A.; Mirocha, J.; Zakowski, P.C.; Zabner, R.; Gaultier, C.R.; et al. Heart transplantation for chagas cardiomyopathy in the united states: Heart transplantation for chagas disease. *Am. J. Transplant.* **2013**, *13*, 3262–3268. [CrossRef] [PubMed]
6. Bacal, F.; Silva, C.P.; Pires, P.V.; Mangini, S.; Fiorelli, A.I.; Stolf, N.G.; Bocchi, E.A. Transplantation for Chagas' disease: An overview of immunosuppression and reactivation in the last two decades. *Clin. Transplant.* **2010**, *24*, E29–E34. [CrossRef] [PubMed]
7. Moreira, M.d.C.V.; Renan Cunha-Melo, J. Chagas disease infection reactivation after heart transplant. *Trop. Med. Infect. Dis.* **2020**, *5*, 106. [CrossRef] [PubMed]
8. Fragata Filho, A.A.; da Silva, M.A.; Boainain, E. Ethiologic treatment of acute and chronic Chagas' disease [corrected]. *São Paulo Med. J. Rev. Paul. Med.* **1995**, *113*, 867–872. [CrossRef] [PubMed]

9. Rassi, A.; Amato Neto, V.; de Siqueira, A.F.; Ferriolli Filho, F.; Amato, V.S.; Rassi Júnior, A. Protective effect of benznidazole against parasite reactivation in patients chronically infected with Trypanosoma cruzi and treated with corticoids for associated diseases. *Rev. Soc. Bras. Med. Trop.* **1999**, *32*, 475–482. [CrossRef] [PubMed]
10. Bacal, F.; Silva, C.P.; Bocchi, E.A.; Pires, P.V.; Moreira, L.F.P.; Issa, V.S.; Moreira, S.A.; das Dores Cruz, F.; Strabelli, T.; Stolf, N.A.G.; et al. Mychophenolate mofetil increased chagas disease reactivation in heart transplanted patients: Comparison between two different protocols. *Am. J. Transplant. Off. J. Am. Soc. Transplant. Am. Soc. Transpl. Surg.* **2005**, *5*, 2017–2021. [CrossRef] [PubMed]
11. Ministerio da Saude. CONITEC. Protocolo Clínico e Diretrizes Terapêuticas Doença de Chagas. 2018. Available online: http://conitec.gov.br/images/Protocolos/Relatorio_PCDT_Doenca_de_Chagas.pdf (accessed on 4 August 2020).
12. Sousa, A.A.; Lobo, M.C.S.G.; Barbosa, R.A.; Bello, V. Chagas seropositive donors in kidney transplantation. *Transplant. Proc.* **2004**, *36*, 868–869. [CrossRef] [PubMed]
13. D'Albuquerque, L.A.C.; Gonzalez, A.M.; Filho, H.L.V.N.; Copstein, J.L.M.; Larrea, F.I.S.; Mansero, J.M.P.; Perón, G.; Ribeiro, M.A.F.; Oliveira e Silva, A. Liver transplantation from deceased donors serologically positive for Chagas disease. *Am. J. Transplant. Off. J. Am. Soc. Transplant. Am. Soc. Transpl. Surg.* **2007**, *7*, 680–684. [CrossRef] [PubMed]
14. de Souza, M.M.; Franco, M.; Almeida, D.R.; Diniz, R.V.; Mortara, R.A.; da Silva, S.; Reis da Silva Patrício, F. Comparative histopathology of endomyocardial biopsies in chagasic and non-chagasic heart transplant recipients. *J. Heart Lung Transplant. Off. Publ. Int. Soc. Heart Transplant.* **2001**, *20*, 534–543. [CrossRef]
15. Gray, E.B.; La Hoz, R.M.; Green, J.S.; Vikram, H.R.; Benedict, T.; Rivera, H.; Montgomery, S.P. Reactivation of Chagas disease among heart transplant recipients in the United States, 2012–2016. *Transpl. Infect. Dis.* **2018**, *20*, e12996. [CrossRef] [PubMed]
16. da Costa, P.A.; Segatto, M.; Durso, D.F.; de Carvalho Moreira, W.J.; Junqueira, L.L.; de Castilho, F.M.; de Andrade, S.A.; Gelape, C.L.; Chiari, E.; Teixeira-Carvalho, A.; et al. Early polymerase chain reaction detection of Chagas disease reactivation in heart transplant patients. *J. Heart Lung Transplant.* **2017**, *36*, 797–805. [CrossRef] [PubMed]
17. Diez, M.; Favaloro, L.; Bertolotti, A.; Burgos, J.M.; Vigliano, C.; Lastra, M.P.; Levin, M.J.; Arnedo, A.; Nagel, C.; Schijman, A.G.; et al. Usefulness of PCR strategies for early diagnosis of Chagas' disease reactivation and treatment follow-up in heart transplantation. *Am. J. Transplant. Off. J. Am. Soc. Transplant. Am. Soc. Transpl. Surg.* **2007**, *7*, 1633–1640. [CrossRef] [PubMed]
18. Schijman, A.G. Molecular diagnosis of Trypanosoma cruzi. *Acta Trop.* **2018**, *184*, 59–66. [CrossRef] [PubMed]
19. Dias, J.C.P.; Ramos, A.N.; Gontijo, E.D.; Luquetti, A.; Shikanai-Yasuda, M.A.; Coura, J.R.; Torres, R.M.; Melo, J.R.d.C.; Almeida, E.A.d.; Oliveira, W.d.; et al. Brazilian consensus on chagas disease, 2015. *Epidemiol. E Serv. Saude Rev. Sist. Unico Saude Bras.* **2016**, *25*, 7–86. [CrossRef] [PubMed]

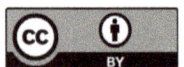

© 2020 by the authors. Licensee MDPI, Basel, Switzerland. This article is an open access article distributed under the terms and conditions of the Creative Commons Attribution (CC BY) license (http://creativecommons.org/licenses/by/4.0/).

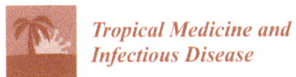 Tropical Medicine and Infectious Disease

Article

Funding for Chagas Disease: A 10-Year (2009–2018) Survey

Leandro S. Sangenito [1], **Marta H. Branquinha** [1] **and André L. S. Santos** [1,2,]*

[1] Laboratório de Estudos Avançados de Microrganismos Emergentes e Resistentes (LEAMER), Departamento de Microbiologia Geral, Instituto de Microbiologia Paulo de Góes (IMPG), Universidade Federal do Rio de Janeiro (UFRJ), Rio de Janeiro 21941-901, Brazil; ibastefano@hotmail.com (L.S.S.); mbranquinha@micro.ufrj.br (M.H.B.)
[2] Programa de Pós-Graduação em Bioquímica (PPGBq), Instituto de Química, Universidade Federal do Rio de Janeiro, Rio de Janeiro 21941-902, Brazil
[*] Correspondence: andre@micro.ufrj.br; Tel.: +55-21-39380366

Received: 24 April 2020; Accepted: 27 May 2020; Published: 1 June 2020

Abstract: Chagas disease was discovered in 1909 by the Brazilian scientist Carlos Chagas. After more than 110 years, many outcomes have been achieved in all research fields; however, Chagas disease remains a serious public health problem, mainly in Latin America, being one of the most neglected tropical diseases in the world. As a neglected disease, it receives very little financial support. Nevertheless, how much is actually spent? With this question in mind, the goal of the present work was to summarize all funding employed by multiple institutions in the Chagas disease field in a 10-year survey. From 2009 to 2018, Chagas disease received only USD 236.31 million, representing 0.67% of the total applied for all neglected diseases in this period. Mostly, the investments are concentrated in basic research (47%) and drug development (42.5%), with the public sector responsible for 74% of all funding, followed by the industry (19%) and philanthropy (7%). Relevantly, NIH (USA) alone accounted for more than half of the total investment. Taking into account that Chagas disease has a great socio-economic impact, it is clear that more investments are needed, especially from endemic countries. Furthermore, coordinated strategies to make better use of resources and incentives for the pharmaceutical industry must be adopted.

Keywords: Chagas disease; human illness; neglected tropical disease; global financing; annual funding; investments

1. Chagas Disease: An Overview

The American trypanosomiasis, or Chagas disease, is listed by the World Health Organization (WHO) as one of the 20 neglected tropical diseases (NTDs) [1,2]. The WHO estimates that 6 to 8 million people are infected with *Trypanosoma cruzi*, the etiologic agent of Chagas disease, and about 12 to 14 thousand deaths are reported every year (4.5 thousand only in Brazil). If left untreated, Chagas disease also can lead to severe digestive and heart system problems over the years [3]. Furthermore, more than 70 million individuals are living in areas with constant risk of transmission. The main form of contagion is through the blood-sucking triatomine insect bite; however, other forms of transmission are also reported, such as blood transfusions or organ/bone marrow transplants without proper control, congenital transmission (mainly in urban and non-endemic areas), laboratory accidents, and orally, by ingesting food or liquids (e.g., açaí berry, palm wine, and sugar cane and guava juices) contaminated with triatomine feces containing infective *T. cruzi* metacyclic trypomastigotes [3,4]. This situation could have been worse if large-scale investments did not begin in the 90 s in order to promote interventions to interrupt the transmission. Important successful examples of multinational collaborations in Latin America must be exalted, such as the Southern Cone, Amazon, Andean and

Central America initiatives. The common goals of these coordinated programs were to eradicate the main triatomine vectors of *T. cruzi* (*Rhodnius prolixus, Triatoma infestans, T. brasiliensis* and *T. dimidiata*) in combination with mandatory serological blood-bank screening [5–8]. Indeed, as vector and blood transfusion transmission has been combated in many countries, the incidence of Chagas disease has dropped substantially over the last decades [9].

Chagas disease is endemic in 21 countries of Latin America (about 6 million cases), but, due to the immigration, it is also reported in developed countries such as United States of America (USA) and some countries in Europe, such as Italy, Spain and France, representing a significant economic burden to the health care systems of these regions [3,10,11] (Figure 1). In Latin America, Argentina, Bolivia, Brazil and Mexico are in the top in terms of prevalence rates, accounting for approximately 70% (4.2 million) of the estimated cases of infected people [4,12].

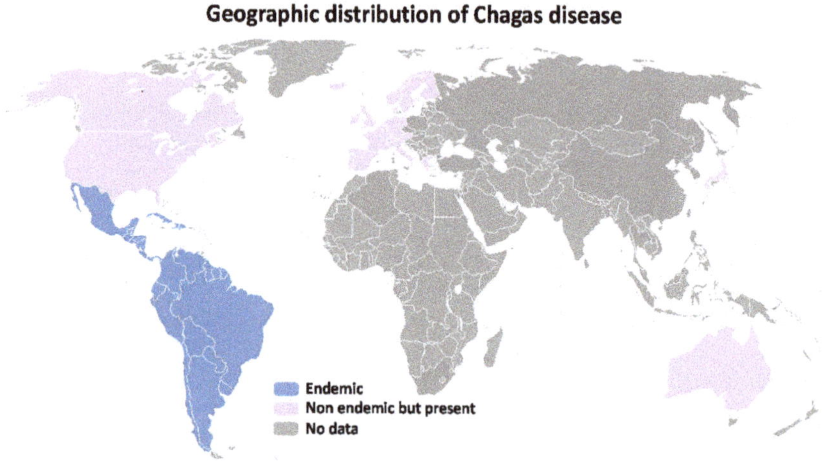

Figure 1. Global distribution showing the countries endemic for Chagas disease, where transmission occurs mainly through insect vector action, as well as the countries that receive infected people from these regions due to the migratory process [3,10,11].

There are several concerns about coping with this disease: besides the lack of an available vaccine, it is estimated that less than 10% of the people in the world affected by Chagas disease are diagnosed and only about 1% have access to specific treatment. The current treatment options, benznidazole and nifurtimox (the latter used in a smaller scale), have doubtful efficacy and require continuous monitoring. Moreover, these compounds present high manufacturing costs and they are extremely toxic, causing several side effects due to the necessity of long-term administration, which may require premature treatment interruption [13,14].

Despite the high morbidity and mortality rates and high costs of hospitalization and treatment, it has been clear that the pharmaceutical sector does not have any serious interest in financing specific research against Chagas disease, as it has for other chronic illness. Unfortunately, it is likely that this scenario has occurred because the population affected by this trypanosomiasis lives in poverty and, therefore, little financial return is expected with the development of diagnostic tests and new chemotherapeutic options. In part, this historical negligence contributes to the increase of disease morbimortality as well as to the spread poverty, and generates more social stigma [2,14–16].

The global impact of Chagas disease can be measured by Disability-Adjusted Life-Years (DALYs), an indicator that takes into account premature deaths and long-term irreversible injuries owing to the disease [17]. Per year, an impressive number, about 700,000, of DALYs has been attributed to Chagas disease, resulting in an overall cost of more than USD 7.2 billion [10,18]. The highest economic impact occurring outside Latin America is attributed to the USA, with an estimated average cost of USD 850 million. Inside Latin America, in Brazil alone, the annual economic losses are estimated at over USD 1.5 billion [10,18]. At the early stages of the disease, the estimated cost per patient is USD 200, but at the chronic symptomatic stage, this value can reach USD 4000 to USD 6000 [19].

For all the reasons mentioned, it is evident that Chagas disease has a huge social and economic global impact. Based on this scenario, it is clear that investments against the disease are extremely necessary. However, how much is actually applied and what is the profile of these investments? In this context, the present work aimed to briefly compile the investments applied to Chagas disease in a 10-year period (2009–2018), as well as the flow of them between the products and the main funders.

2. Data Collection for the Survey

This work was elaborated by compiling information collected from the repository of investment data provided by the G-FINDER project, conducted by Policy Cures Research, a not-for-profit global health think tank funded by the Bill & Melinda Gates Foundation [20]. The G-FINDER project groups annual funding data on neglected diseases provided by hundreds of institutions of governmental, private and philanthropic sectors. The survey was conducted from 2009 to 2018 (10 years) considering funding applied exclusively on Chagas disease, thus excluding investments in research and development (R&D) for multiple trypanosomiasis (Chagas disease, leishmaniasis and sleeping sickness). The year 2019 was not included in this work as data collection has not yet been completed. Pharmaceutical industry funding is presented aggregated for confidentiality reasons. For a better comparison of annual changes, funding data of all years were adjusted for the 2018 inflation rate and presented in US dollars (USD) to eliminate artefactual effects caused by inflation and exchange rate fluctuations.

3. Funds Applied to Chagas Disease over 10 Years

According to the data collected in the survey, the total amount of funds for R&D on neglected diseases reached almost USD 35 billion in a period of 10 years (2009–2018). The global investment in neglected diseases changed little over these years, with the exception of the year 2018, when the investment brand passed the USD 4 billion mark (Table 1). The majority of the global investments (USD 25 billion or 71.71%) were directed to only three diseases: AIDS, tuberculosis and malaria. In fact, this proportion is expected, since this "evil triad" corresponded to almost 276 million registered cases worldwide in 2018 (37.9 million of AIDS, 10 million of tuberculosis and 228 million of malaria) [21–23]. In 2018, the number of malaria deaths stood at 405 thousand (of these, an incredible 272 thousand were deaths of children under 5 years of age). The African region continues to carry a disproportionately high share of the global malaria burden, with 93% of malaria cases and 94% of malaria deaths [21]. Similarly, the African region accounts for more than two-thirds (25.7 million) of all people living with AIDS. The remaining (12.2 million) cases are spread across the world, but mainly in Eastern Europe and Central Asia. In 2018, 770 thousand people died from AIDS-related causes [22]. Tuberculosis is a treatable and curable disease. Even so, 1.5 million people died in 2018 (including 251 thousand people co-infected with HIV). A terrifying number of child deaths, 205 thousand, was also reported due to the tuberculosis (including among children infected with HIV). Tuberculosis is present in every part of the world. Therefore, the largest number of new cases in 2018 occurred in the South-East Asian region, with 44% of new cases, followed by the African region, with 24% of new cases and the Western Pacific with 18% [23]. Consequently, the high investment earmarked for this triad is easily justified by, collectively, the large number of cases worldwide, the global spread of the diseases and both morbidity and mortality rates, which mainly affect poor and developing countries as well as specific groups living in developed countries.

Table 1. Investments in neglected diseases over 10 years [20].

Investments in Neglected Diseases in 10 Years (USD in Million *)												
Diseases	2009	2010	2011	2012	2013	2014	2015	2016	2017	2018	Total	%
Neglected Diseases	3595	3416	3364	3469	3348	3337	3282	3437	3681	4055	34,984	100
Chagas Diseases	19.31	23.3	27.03	35.28	28.3	21.65	19.15	23.4	17.94	20.95	236.31	0.67

* Adjusted values for 2018 inflation.

Unfortunately, investments in Chagas disease do not reflect the reality described above. In 10 years, the amount invested was USD 236.31 million, only 0.67% of the total applied for neglected diseases overall (Table 1). Both the number of infected people and the deaths associated with Chagas disease are inaccurate and probably underestimated [4]. For example, Chagas disease received USD 20.95 millionin 2018, which represents only from USD 2.6 to USD 3.5 per infected person and from USD 1496 thousand to USD1745 thousand per death. The investments combined for malaria, tuberculosis and AIDS in 2018 summed to USD 2.8 billion, representing about USD 10.2 per infected person (2.9 to 3.9 higher than for Chagas disease) and USD 1155 thousand per death (USD 340 to USD 590 less than Chagas disease). The "evil triad" has a higher lethality rate than Chagas disease; for this reason, the amount employed by death ends up being lower in view of the greater number of deaths. In this comparison, despite the lower lethality rate, the chronic form of Chagas disease is considered a disabling illness responsible for the most significant morbidity and mortality among parasitic diseases, in addition to great social stigma [4]. Indeed, as already mentioned, 700,000 DALYs have been attributed to Chagas disease each year (while DALYs for malaria in Latin America were estimated at 111,000), with a global cost for health systems exceeding the USD 7 billion mark, which reinforces the constant need for attention to this illness [2,4,12]. Therefore, appropriated investments in health care interventions should be framed in terms of the long-term savings to healthcare systemsas well as the economy [24].

In another comparison, other trypanosomatid diseases, such as leishmaniasis and sleeping sickness (or HAT, human African trypanosomiasis), also received much more funding in 10 years than Chagas disease: respectively, USD 503 million and USD 425 million. Leishmaniasis is endemic in approximately 98 countries worldwide, but especially located in Latin America, East Africa and Southeast Asia, with 14 million people directly affected by the three forms of the disease (cutaneous, mucocutaneous and visceral). By far, visceral leishmaniasis is the most important form, because it causes the most severe disease, with 200–400 thousand cases per year with 10%–20% mortality [25]. Moreover, leishmaniasis is also of great importance in the context of veterinary medicine: dogs have great domestic appeal as well as being the main reservoirs for several *Leishmania* species. Therefore, it should be noted that this dichotomy is responsible for part of the USD 38.87 million investment destined to the disease in 2018 [26]. HAT, on the other hand, is a more restricted disease, affecting mainly African countries such as the Democratic Republic of the Cong, which is responsible for 70% of the cases reported in the last 10 years. Although fewer than 977 cases were reported in 2018 in endemic countries, HAT is still a public health problem in endemic regions, receiving USD 50.63 million of investments in the same year [27,28]. In general, investments destined for Chagas disease summed to around the USD 20 million mark. Three years stood out: 2011, with USD 27.03 million, 2012, with USD 35.28 million, and 2013 with USD 28.3 million. Notably, in 2012, the percentage directed to American trypanosomiasis managed to slightly pass the mark of 1% of the total applied for neglected diseases in the same year (Table 1). In 2008, Chagas disease received an investment of around USD 18 million. It is interesting to note that, even with the huge world economic crisis of 2008 [29], investments in Chagas disease continued to rise, reaching theirpeak in 2012, when they started to stabilize (Table 1).

R&D funding for Chagas disease is largely concentrated in basic research (47%) and development/repositioning of drugs (42.5%). On a second level, the development of diagnostics and vaccines accounts for only 10% of funding flow. All remaining products (biologics, vector control and others) received less than 1%. In 2009 and 2010, basic research received about three times the total applied for the development of new therapies. Thereafter, the flow of financing for drug products received an extraordinary increase in 2011 (up to USD 6.31 million, which corresponds to 114.1%), even surpassing the basic research funding in the subsequent years 2012, 2013, 2014 and 2015. In 2017, the funds for drugs went back to the level of earlier years due to many cuts (Table 2). In part, the Brazilian Support Foundation for Research in the State of São Paulo (FAPESP) dropped out of the top main funders because no funding was reported for Chagas disease R&D in 2017, due to the steep cuts in Brazilian public agencies' spending. In 2018, a notable increase in funding for drug R&D (up USD 6.87 million, which corresponds to 154.7%), occurred again, as a result of record high industry investment and the Mundo Sano Foundation's USD 1.8 million grant to the Drugs for Neglected Diseases *initiative* (DND*i*) for pediatric benznidazole to treat Chagas disease.

Table 2. Chagas disease R&D funding [20].

Chagas Disease R&D Funding in 10 Years (USD in Million *)											
Areas	2009	2010	2011	2012	2013	2014	2015	2016	2017	2018	Total by Product
Basic Research	13.47	14.07	11.74	14.26	9.82	8.14	8.12	12.06	11.48	7.78	110.94
Drugs	4.38	5.53	11.84	17.54	16.41	11.64	9.21	8.02	4.44	11.31	100.32
Diagnostics	0.9	2.79	3.15	3.01	1.63	1.24	1.09	2.0	1.67	1.75	19.23
Vaccines	0.53	0.86	0.26	0.26	0.21	0.42	0.63	0.92	0.26	0.02	4.37
Biologics	NA	0.02	0.01	NA	NA	0.02	<0.01	0.26	0.02	0.02	0.35
Vector Control	<0.01	NA	NA	0.01	0.03	NA	NA	0.06	0.05	0.04	0.2
Other	0.02	0.01	0.01	0.18	0.2	0.17	0.09	0.04	0.02	0.03	0.77
Total by Disease	19.31	23.3	27.03	35.28	28.3	21.65	19.15	23.4	17.94	20.95	

* Adjusted values for 2018 inflation; NA, not applied.

The responsibility for investing in Chagas disease falls mainly on the shoulders of the public sector. In 10 years, governmental institutions were responsible for 74% of total funding (USD 174.77 million). In the second place, industry funding reached 19% of total funding (USD 44.44 million), followed by philanthropic institutions with 7% (USD 17.1 million) (Figure 2A). If only the funding from public sector is taken into account, 60.9% (USD 106.48 million) was applied to basic research. This amount represents 96% of total funding designated for basic research in 10 years, demonstrating the great dependence of this type of research on the public sector. Here, we emphasize that the investment in basic research includes all investment for Chagas disease/*T. cruzi*. However, although much research deals with the pathogen that causes the disease, this research may not have a direct influence on combating the disease itself. The public sector also significantly funds drug development/repositioning, designating 26.5% (USD 46.38 million) of its total investments. Although the public sector allocates "only" about a quarter of its entire investment in drug products, this total, USD 46.38 million, represents about 46.2% of the total investment in drugs over 10 years. Another 44.1% (USD 44.25 million) of the total funds for drug products came from the aggregate industry. It is also interesting to note that this portion basically represents the whole private sector investment. The remaining 9.67% of total drug funds (USD 9.7 million) were donated by philanthropic organizations, which also represented the main destination of resources (56.7%) from this type of funder. Finally, public agencies were also responsible for funding 87.3% of total investments in diagnosis. The remaining funds (12.6%, USD 2.43 million) came almost entirely from philanthropy (Figure 2B).

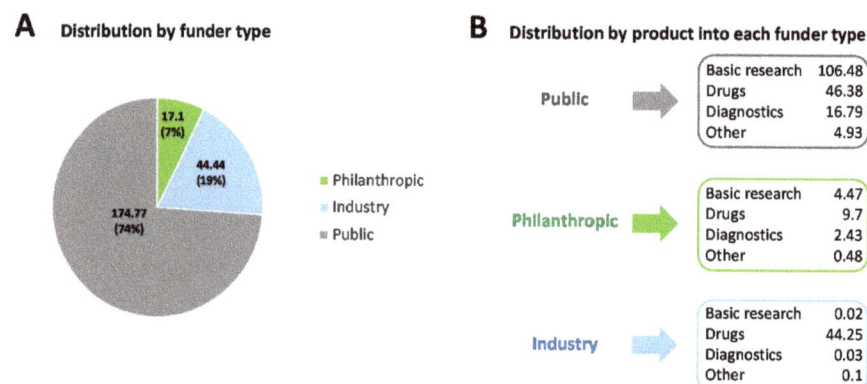

Figure 2. (**A**) Funds invested in Chagas disease for 10 years by the three main investment sectors. (**B**) Funds from the three main investment sectors distributed by product each type [20]. The values are adjusted for 2018 inflation and are expressed in US million dollars.

In a list of more than 50 R&D funders of all types, the top 20 accounted for 96.8% of all R&D funding for Chagas disease over 10 years. However, the top three funders alone—the US NIH, industry, and the Wellcome Trust—provided nearly three-quarters (USD 180.26 million, 76.3%) of all funding (Table 3). If the funds over 10 years are separated by geographic regions, excluding the aggregate industrial sector, investors in North America are responsible for the majority (USD 124.3 million) of R&D financing of Chagas disease. Within these, the public sector of the American government, represented by the NIH, was solely responsible for investing USD 119.79 million of that amount, with the remainder practically coming from Mexico (Figure 3A, Table 3). Interestingly, Europe is responsible for the second-largest portion of all investments in Chagas disease, about USD 36.7 million. Within this, USD 17.84 million (48.6%) was destined to basic research, followed by USD 15.32 million (41.74%) for drug development/repositioning and USD 2.91 million (7.93%) for diagnostic products. This huge investment is due to the great contribution of the philanthropic institution the Wellcome Trust, the European commission, and Institute Pasteur, which reflects the European concern with Latin American immigrants who arrive infected with *T. cruzi* and become a public health problem for their governments (Figure 3A, Table 3) [3,30]. Indeed, Basile and coworkers [31] estimated the number of *T. cruzi*-infected immigrants living in Europeas ranging between 68,318 and 123,078, with 4290 confirmed cases, 94%–96% remaining undiagnosed. This scenario stimulated several meetings to address the problem, leading to recommendations, formation of coordinated working groups and adoption of various control measures [3,30]. Finally, South America, the region with the vast majority of cases, is the geographic region providing thethird-most R&D funds (Figure 3). This fact should be seriously reviewed, since Chagas disease is mainly a South American problem. Therefore, it is unacceptable that South America spends less to combat the illness than Europe, despite the fact that the gross domestic product of some South American countries is comparable to some European countries [32].

The top 10 countries that invest in Chagas disease are listed in Figure 3B. By far, the USA appears as the major funder, contributing USD 121.45 million. In second place is the United Kingdom (UK), contributing USD 16.45 million, where 97.4% (USD 16.03 million) came from the generosity of the philanthropic institution the Wellcome Trust. Brazil appears in the third position, followed very closely by France, Argentina and Chile (Figure 3B, Table 3). It is terrifying to note that Bolivia, one of the main countries in terms of cases and risk of infection [4,12], does not figure in the list of the main funders of R&D to control American trypanosomiasis, perhaps due to the lack of participation of the country's agencies in providing data.

5. Conclusions

The present work summarized the investments applied to Chagas disease over a period of 10 years. As we have seen, little funding has been directed towards to this specific parasitic illness when compared to other neglected diseases. For a human disease that is responsible annually for about 700,000 DALYs, with an economic impact of more than USD 7 billion, receiving just 0.67% (USD 236.3 million) of the total budget for neglected diseases (considering the period from 2009 to 2018) is unacceptable and meaningless. Therefore, allocating more funds to fight Chagas disease is urgently necessary in terms of saving lives, restoring quality of life and reducing the economic impact coming from health care systems.

Regarding Chagas disease, clearly, funding depends much more on the public sector (74%) than on other areas (private and philanthropic). However, public agencies in Latin American countries contribute very little compared to NIH-USA, a situation that needs to be reviewed. In addition, development agencies, governments and the Chagas disease community must work in unison to ensure that the (scarce) resources are well applied. In parallel, there is a need to adopt strategies and market incentives to attract the pharmaceutical industry more to the Chagas disease cause, since the sector contributed only USD 44.4 million over 10 years. Other relevant issues to be addressed include the low investment in important tools such as diagnostics, vaccines and vector control, which together received just 10% of the total budget, with the remaining equally distributed in basic research and drug development/repositioning.

Finally, we hope that this survey helps to support the work of many other groups in the Chagas disease community, facilitating decision-making and even more effective application of the available resources.

Author Contributions: L.S.S., M.H.B. and A.L.S.S. participated in the conceptualization, formal analysis, data curation, writing, reviewing of the manuscript. All authors have read and agreed to the published version of the manuscript.

Funding: This work was supported by grants from Fundação Carlos Chagas Filho de Amparo à Pesquisa do Estado do Rio de Janeiro (FAPERJ), Conselho Nacional de Desenvolvimento Científico e Tecnológico (CNPq) and Coordenação de Aperfeiçoamento de Pessoal de Nível Superior (CAPES, Financial code-001).

Conflicts of Interest: The authors declare that they have no conflict of interest.

References

1. World Health Organization. 2020. Available online: https://www.who.int/neglected_diseases/diseases/en/ (accessed on 20 March 2020).
2. Crager, S.E.; Price, M. Prizes and Parasites: Incentive Models for Addressing Chagas Disease. *J. Law Med. Ethics* **2009**, *37*, 292–304. [CrossRef] [PubMed]
3. Lidani, K.C.F.; Andrade, F.A.; Bavia, L.; Damasceno, F.S.; Beltrame, M.H.; Messias-Reason, I.J.; Sandri, T.L. Chagas disease: From discovery to a worldwide health problem. *Front. Public Health* **2019**, *2*, 166. [CrossRef] [PubMed]
4. Pinheiro, E.; Brum-Soares, L.; Reis, R.; Cubides, J.C. Chagas disease: Review of needs, neglect, and obstacles to treatment access in Latin America. *Rev. Soc. Bras. Med. Trop.* **2017**, *3*, 296–300. [CrossRef] [PubMed]
5. Schofield, C.J.; Dias, J.C. The Southern Cone Initiative against Chagas disease. *Adv. Parasitol.* **1999**, *42*, 1–27. [CrossRef]
6. Guzmán-Bracho, C. Epidemiology of Chagas disease in Mexico: An update. *Trends Parasitol.* **2001**, *8*, 372–376. [CrossRef]
7. Guhl, F.; Restrepo, M.; Angulo, V.M.; Antunes, C.M.; Campbell-Lendrum, D.; Davies, C.R. Lessons from a national survey of Chagas disease transmission risk in Colombia. *Trends Parasitol.* **2005**, *6*, 259–562. [CrossRef]
8. Hashimoto, K.; Schofield, C.J. Elimination of *Rhodnius prolixus* in Central America. *Parasites Vectors* **2012**, *5*, 45. [CrossRef]
9. Chuit, R.; Meiss, R.; Salvatella, R.; Altcheh, J.; Freilij, H. Epidemiology of Chagas Disease. In *Chagas Disease*; Springer: Cham, Switzerland, 2019; Volume 351, pp. 91–109. [CrossRef]

10. Lee, B.Y.; Bacon, K.M.; Bottazzi, M.E.; Hotez, P.J. Global economic burden of Chagas disease: A computational simulation model. *Lancet Infect. Dis.* **2013**, *4*, 342–348. [CrossRef]
11. World Health Organization. Chagas disease in Latin America: An epidemiological update based on 2010 estimates. *Wkl. Epidemiol. Rec. (WER)* **2015**, *6*, 33–44. Available online: http://www.who.int/wer/2015/wer9006.pdf (accessed on 21 March 2020).
12. World Health Organization. Investing to overcome the global impact of neglected tropical diseases: Third WHO report on neglected diseases. *Libr. Cat. Publ. Data* **2015**, *2*, 75–81. Available online: http://apps.who.int/iris/bitstream/10665/152781/1/9789241564861_eng.pdf?ua=1 (accessed on 21 March 2020).
13. Sales, P.A.; Molina, I.; Fonseca, M.S.M.; Sánchez-Montalvá, A.; Salvador, F.; Corrêa-Oliveira, R.; Carneiro, C.M. Experimental and clinical treatment of Chagas disease: A review. *Am. J. Trop. Med. Hyg.* **2017**, *5*, 1289–1303. [CrossRef] [PubMed]
14. Drugs for Neglected Diseases Initiative. 2019. Available online: https://www.dndi.org/wp-content/uploads/2019/09/Factsheet2019_ChagasDisease.pdf (accessed on 21 March 2020).
15. Bhutta, Z.A.; Sommerfeld, J.; Lassi, Z.S.; Salam, R.A.; Das, J.K. Global burden, distribution, and interventions for infectious diseases of poverty. *Infect. Dis. Poverty* **2014**, *3*, 21. [CrossRef] [PubMed]
16. Sangenito, L.S.; da Silva, S.V.; d'Avila-Levy, C.M.; Branquinha, M.H.; Santos, A.L.S.; Oliveira, S.S.C. Leishmaniasis and Chagas disease—neglected tropical diseases: Treatment updates. *Curr. Top. Med. Chem.* **2019**, *3*, 174–177. [CrossRef] [PubMed]
17. Dias, L.C.; Dessoy, M.A.; Silva, J.J.N.; Thiemann, O.H.; Oliva, G.; Andricopulo, A.D. Chemotherapy of Chagas' disease: State of the art and perspectives for the development of new drugs. *Quim. Nova* **2009**, *9*, 2444–2457. [CrossRef]
18. Ferreira, L.G.; de Oliveira, M.T.; Andricopulo, A.D. Advances and progress in Chagas disease drug discovery. *Curr. Top. Med. Chem.* **2016**, *20*, 2290–2302. [CrossRef]
19. Abuhab, A.; Trindade, E.; Aulicino, G.B.; Fujii, S.; Bocchi, E.A.; Bacal, F. Chagas' cardiomyopathy: The economic burden of an expensive and neglected disease. *Int. J. Cardiol.* **2013**, *168*, 2375–2380. [CrossRef]
20. G-Finder Project. Available online: https://gfinderdata.policycuresresearch.org/ (accessed on 29 March 2020).
21. Malaria Fact Sheets. 2020. Available online: https://www.who.int/news-room/feature-stories/detail/world-malaria-report-2019 (accessed on 30 April 2020).
22. AIDS Fact Sheets. 2020. Available online: https://www.who.int/news-room/fact-sheets/detail/hiv-aids (accessed on 1 May 2020).
23. Tuberculosis Fact Sheets. 2020. Available online: https://www.who.int/en/news-room/fact-sheets/detail/tuberculosis (accessed on 1 May 2020).
24. Echeverría, L.E.; Marcus, R.; Novick, G.; Sosa-Estani, S.; Ralston, K.; Zaidel, E.; Forsyth, C.; Ribeiro, L.P.; Mendoza, I.; Falconi, M.L.; et al. WHF IASC Roadmap on Chagas Disease. *Glob. Heart* **2020**, *1*, 26. [CrossRef]
25. Leishmaniasis Fact Sheets. 2020. Available online: https://www.who.int/news-room/fact-sheets/detail/leishmaniasis (accessed on 2 May 2020).
26. Dantas-Torres, F.; Miró, G.; Baneth, G.; Bourdeau, P.; Breitschwerdt, E.; Capelli, G.; Cardoso, L.; Day, M.J.; Dobler, G.; Ferrer, L.; et al. Canine Leishmaniasis Control in the Context of One Health. *Emerg. Infect. Dis.* **2019**, *12*, 1–4. [CrossRef]
27. Sleeping Sickness Fact Sheets. 2020. Available online: https://www.who.int/news-room/fact-sheets/detail/trypanosomiasis-human-african-(sleeping-sickness) (accessed on 2 May 2020).
28. Gao, J.M.; Qian, Z.Y.; Hide, G.; Lai, D.H.; Lun, Z.R.; Wu, Z.D. Human African trypanosomiasis: The current situation in endemic regions and the risks for non-endemic regions from imported cases. *Parasitology* **2020**, *27*, 1–28. [CrossRef]
29. World Health Organization. Available online: https://www.who.int/topics/financial_crisis/financialcrisis_report_200902.pdf (accessed on 1 April 2020).
30. Liu, Q.; Zhou, X.N. Preventing the transmission of American trypanosomiasis and its spread into non-endemic countries. *Infect. Dis. Poverty* **2015**, *4*, 60. [CrossRef]
31. Basile, I.; Jansà, J.M.; Carlier, Y.; Salamanca, D.D.; Angheben, A.; Bartoloni, A.; Seixas, J.; Van Gool, T.; Canavate, C.; Flores-Chavez, M.; et al. Chagas disease in European countries: The challenge of a surveillance system. *Euro Surveill.* **2011**, *16*, 19968. [CrossRef] [PubMed]

Table 3. Top 20 funders in Chagas disease [20].

Top 20 Funders in Chagas Disease (USD in Million *)			
1. US NIH	119.79	11. Brazilian FAPESP	2.45
2. Aggregate Industry	44.44	12. French IRD	2.16
3. Wellcome Trust	16.03	13. Mundo Sano Foundation	1.85
4. European Commission	8.9	14. Carlos III Health Institute	1.27
5. Chilean FONDECYT	6.04	15. LAFEPE	1.25
6. Colombian Colciencias	4.85	16. Brazilian FAPEMIG	1.14
7. Institute Pasteur	4.54	17. Brazilian BNDES	1.11
8. Argentinian MINCYT	4.4	18. French ANR	1.04
9. Brazilian DECIT	3.15	19. Argentinian CONICET	0.93
10. Mexican CONACYT	2.48	20. Gates Foundation	0.83

* Adjusted values for 2018 inflation.

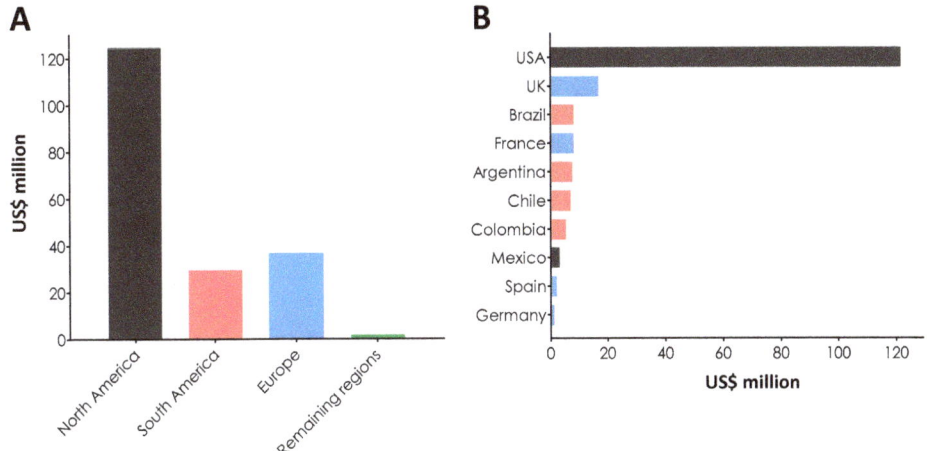

Figure 3. (**A**) Funds for Chagas disease from the main geographic regions. (**B**) Fractioned funds by each country. The colors are correlated with each geographic region in (**B**). The data in (**A**) and (**B**) refer to investments coming from the public sector and philanthropic organizations in each region, thus excluding the private sector, which has headquarters in different countries. The values are adjusted for 2018 inflation and are expressed in USD in million. Note that the countries are grouped by their geographic regions and not by the origin of the spoken language (like the Latin American countries); in this way, Mexico is found in North America [20].

The major change in the last fifteen years in the Chagas disease landscape has been the appearance of new investigators and initiatives from the pharmaceutical industry, academic groups, and consortia, encouraging and promoting further R&D in the area [33]. In future years, global financial contributions against Chagas disease will also come from a new partner. At the end of 2019, the international center for the Purchase of Medicines against AIDS, malaria and tuberculosis (UNITAID), an entity created by Brazil, Chile, France, Norway and UK, announced that it will contribute, for the first time, USD 20 million over four years [34]. The idea is to develop strategies and tools to improve prevention and diagnosis, reduce congenital infection, and provide faster treatments and drug formulations with fewer side effects than the nitroderivatives. The expectation of the entity, which is also a partner of

WHO, is that research institutions of excellence in more than one country will establish new consortia to seek solutions. Indeed, collaborative strategies between several health and research institutions, such as the DND*i*, are a smart bet, which save time and costs and can produce relevant results [16]. Therefore, they must always be considered.

4. Topics to Be Addressed on Chagas Disease Funding

For an illness surrounded by stigma, affecting millions, funding for Chagas disease R&D is far from ideal. Although the last 15 years have seen considerable evolution, there are still several issues to be worked on to overcome the problems associated with limited treatment [4,33]. New advances in R&D from recent clinical trials have been made in the last decade; however, it is urgent to review the current evidence and define future research priorities. A focused and collaborative effort from the entire research community would ensure the development of appropriate and efficacious anti-*T. cruzi* drugs [24]. Collaborative efforts are also welcome for developing other products and pursuing important strategies. For instance, vaccine candidates for Chagas disease are at the pre-clinical stage [35], representing a future front in the battle. Moreover, it is also crucial to scale efforts up to provide easier access to diagnostic testing and medical therapy for chagasic patients. Finally, the designation of resources to triatomine vector control was a rational and the cost-effective approach to drastically reduce the incidence of the disease, but continuation of these public health programs is needed to maintain success [2,36]. While increasing spending may cause acute strain on research budgets, it is clear that improving preventative efforts on Chagas disease can effectively reduce this spending over time [24].

Usually, development agencies focus their spending majority on operational and field research, not R&D. This statement also appears at the basic level of global health planning with the premise that new technologies would divert attention and funding away from real concerns [36]. Global health agencies, including the WHO, do not consider R&D a core indicator that the global community prioritizes. They take the position that scarce funds should be primarily spent on traditional public health issues such as infrastructure, the workforce, health data and health services. This is extremely unfounded and unhelpful since promising innovation does not compete with program health funding. The initial cost of R&D, which seems high during the innovation process, becomes smaller and smaller over decades of use, especially when set against the saving of lives and health resources [36]. The imperative for public health programs was to prioritize the resources already available, employing low-cost tools for many neglected health problems (more than 95% of drugs on the WHO's Essential Medicines List were older off-patent drugs) [37]. Moreover, pharmaceutical companies seek firstly profit maximization, not global public health improvement. To contextualize, of the 1556 new compounds brought to market between the period from 1975 to 2004, only 20 (1.28%) were for neglected diseases, and none of them for Chagas disease [38]. Even with little investment in innovation, it is no surprise that all of these 20 compounds were developed with public-sector involvement [2]. It is critical that the international community take it upon themselves to address the predictable gap in R&D (that disproportionately affects developing countries) conducted by the pharmaceutical industry. However, the public sectors also cannot exempt themselves from responsibility and must promote actions that maximize results as well as encourage the private sector to support the cause.

To address the structural R&D gap, coordinated strategies should be employed between global health and development agencies in order to produce new tools and treatments for Chagas disease. For this, the maintenance of a medical R&D agenda driven by Chagas disease needs is crucial, besides serious international and local financing to support this R&D, not just for traditional operational and health systems research. Governments should also cautiously promote market-based incentives that seek to stimulate pharmaceutical R&D. It is also important to rapidly increase innovation expertise (with open access to the resultant knowledge) in order to achieve effective R&D prioritization and smart funding decisions. Moreover, all subjects of the equation need to engage far more closely with each other, to secure better sequencing of their activities and a better strategic alignment between what the Chagas disease community needs and what the science community does [2,24,36].

32. World Population Review: GDP Ranked by Country. 2020. Available online: https://worldpopulationreview.com/countries/countries-by-gdp/ (accessed on 8 May 2020).
33. Chatelain, E. Chagas Disease Drug Discovery: Toward a New Era. *J. Biomol. Screen.* **2015**, *1*, 22–35. [CrossRef] [PubMed]
34. Brazil, Ministry of Health. Available online: https://www.saude.gov.br/noticias/agencia-saude/46058-brasil-emplaca-maior-investimento-mundial-contra-doenca-de-chagas (accessed on 13 April 2020).
35. Beaumier, C.; Gillespie, P.; Strych, U.; Hayward, T.; Hotez, P.J.; Bottazzi, M.E. Status of vaccine research and development of vaccines for CD. *Vaccine* **2016**, *34*, 2996–3000. [CrossRef] [PubMed]
36. Moran, M. The Grand Convergence: Closing the Divide between Public Health Funding and Global Health Needs. *PLoS Biol.* **2016**, *3*, e1002363. [CrossRef]
37. Saez, C. WHO Reviews Its Essential Medicines List; Some New Candidates Under Patent. Intellectual Property Watch. Available online: https://www.ip-watch.org/2015/04/21/who-reviews-its-essential-medicines-list-some-new-candidates-under-patent/ (accessed on 9 May 2020).
38. Moran, M.; Guzman, J.; Ropars, A.L.; McDonald, A.; Jameson, N.; Omune, B.; Ryan, S.; Wu, L. Neglected disease research and development: How much are we really spending? *PLoS Med.* **2009**, *2*, e30. [CrossRef]

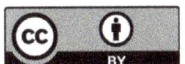

© 2020 by the authors. Licensee MDPI, Basel, Switzerland. This article is an open access article distributed under the terms and conditions of the Creative Commons Attribution (CC BY) license (http://creativecommons.org/licenses/by/4.0/).

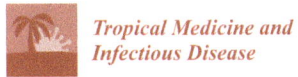

Article

Elucidating the Mechanism of *Trypanosoma cruzi* Acquisition by Triatomine Insects: Evidence from a Large Field Survey of *Triatoma infestans*

Aaron W. Tustin [1], Ricardo Castillo-Neyra [2,3], Laura D. Tamayo [2], Renzo Salazar [2], Katty Borini-Mayorí [2] and Michael Z. Levy [2,3,*]

[1] Department of Environmental Health Sciences, Johns Hopkins Bloomberg School of Public Health, Baltimore, MD 21205, USA; aarontustin2@gmail.com
[2] Zoonotic Disease Research Lab, One Health Unit, School of Public Health and Administration, Universidad Peruana Cayetano Heredia, Lima, Lima Province 15102, Peru; cricardo@upenn.edu (R.C.-N.); laura.tamayo@upch.pe (L.D.T.); rendaths@gmail.com (R.S.); yttakbm@gmail.com (K.B.-M.)
[3] Department of Biostatistics, Epidemiology & Informatics, Perelman School of Medicine of the University of Pennsylvania, Philadelphia, PA 19104, USA
* Correspondence: mzlevy@pennmedicine.upenn.edu; Tel.: +1-215-746-8131

Received: 25 March 2020; Accepted: 26 May 2020; Published: 1 June 2020

Abstract: Blood-sucking triatomine bugs transmit the protozoan parasite *Trypanosoma cruzi*, the etiologic agent of Chagas disease. We measured the prevalence of *T. cruzi* infection in 58,519 *Triatoma infestans* captured in residences in and near Arequipa, Peru. Among bugs from infected colonies, *T. cruzi* prevalence increased with stage from 12% in second instars to 36% in adults. Regression models demonstrated that the probability of parasite acquisition was roughly the same for each developmental stage. Prevalence increased by 5.9% with each additional stage. We postulate that the probability of acquiring the parasite may be related to the number of feeding events. Transmission of the parasite does not appear to be correlated with the amount of blood ingested during feeding. Similarly, other hypothesized transmission routes such as coprophagy fail to explain the observed pattern of prevalence. Our results could have implications for the feasibility of late-acting control strategies that preferentially kill older insects.

Keywords: *Trypanosoma cruzi*; *Triatoma infestans*; Chagas disease; parasite prevalence; coprophagy

1. Introduction

Trypanosoma cruzi, the protozoan parasite that causes Chagas disease, is transmitted to humans via the feces of blood-sucking triatomine insects (Hemiptera: Reduviidae) such as *Triatoma infestans*, the major vector of Chagas disease in much of South America [1]. Triatomines pass through five nymphal instar stages before becoming adults. All triatomine stages are at risk for acquiring *T. cruzi* because they all ingest blood meals. Insects may also become infected when they engage in behaviors such as coprophagy [2]. Once acquired, infection with *T. cruzi* is persistent [3]. Therefore, in well-stablished colonies with stable transmission patterns, *T. cruzi* prevalence is expected to increase monotonically with the insects' developmental stage. The general shape (e.g., linear, exponential, logarithmic) of the rising prevalence curve may give clues as to the method of transmission. With respect to Chagas disease control, it may be important to ascertain the shape of this relationship between *T. cruzi* prevalence and stage.

In this report we show the stage-prevalence of *T. cruzi* in a large sample of *T. infestans* captured during vector control and surveillance activities in Arequipa, Peru. These data allow us to test three hypotheses of *T. cruzi* acquisition by triatomines. Our first hypothesis, hereafter called the Blood

Hypothesis, is that the probability of infection with *T. cruzi* depends upon the amount of blood ingested. Observations of laboratory-reared insects indicate that the quantity of blood ingested by *T. infestans* increases rapidly and nonlinearly with stage [4] Thus, if the Blood Hypothesis is correct, there might be a rapid nonlinear rise in *T. cruzi* prevalence with stage (Figure 1A). A second possibility is that an insect's risk of infection depends upon the number of opportunities to acquire the parasite (Bites Hypothesis), rather than the amount of blood ingested. Under this hypothesis, *T. cruzi* prevalence among instars might rise in a roughly linear fashion with stage (Figure 1B), as all nymphs probably take roughly equal numbers of bites.

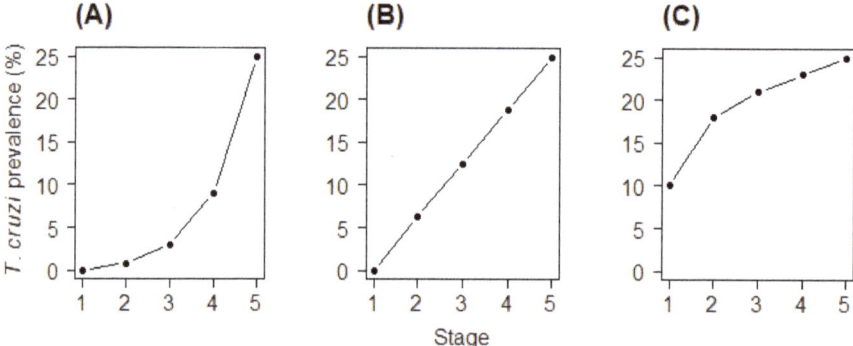

Figure 1. Hypothetical shapes of the relationship between triatomine stage and prevalence of infection with *Trypanosoma cruzi* under three hypotheses. (**A**) Acquisition of the parasite depends upon the quantity of blood ingested (Blood Hypothesis); (**B**) Parasite acquisition depends upon the number of exposure opportunities (Bites Hypothesis); (**C**) Early instar nymphs frequently acquire the parasite via coprophagy, while older instars acquire the parasite at a lower rate via ingestion of blood from mammalian hosts (Coprophagy Hypothesis). Note: the scale of the vertical axis is for illustrative purpose only and does not correspond to actual data; rather, panels (**A**) through (**C**) demonstrate three different theoretical shapes that could each produce 25% prevalence in fifth instars.

The third hypothesis is that triatomines frequently acquire *T. cruzi* via coprophagy (Coprophagy Hypothesis). Triatomines ingest small amounts of feces of older insects in order to acquire bacterial symbionts necessary for digestion of blood meals [5]. Presumably, it is the early instars that ingest feces, as nymphs of some species fail to mature in the absence of symbionts [6]. An isolated experiment has suggested that *T. infestans* may also acquire *T. cruzi* by this route [2]. If parasite transmission via coprophagy is common under field conditions, then *T. cruzi* prevalence may increase relatively quickly among first and second instars, followed by a less rapid increase in older nymphs that acquire the parasite only via blood feeding (Figure 1C).

2. Materials and Methods

Between 2008 and 2014, workers from the Arequipa Ministry of Health and the Universidad Peruana Cayetano Heredia/University of Pennsylvania (UPCH/Penn) Zoonotic Disease Research Laboratory collected triatomines from urban and peri-urban households in and around the city of Arequipa. Located at 2300 m above sea level in an arid zone, Arequipa is the second largest city in Perú, home to 1,008,290 people [7]. Since the 1960s, the population has been growing rapidly due to an influx of immigrants, most of whom have settled on hillsides in the periphery of the city. These settlements are characterized by poorly built housing, mostly constructed with volcanic stone and bricks without mortar, where there is a greater presence of food animals such as guinea pigs or chickens [8]. On the other hand, closer to the center are the oldest neighborhoods (dating back to the late 19th and early 20th centuries), which are inhabited by people with a higher socioeconomic status [9]. The prevalence of *Triatoma infestans*-infested houses between these two types of zones are different: Households in hillside neighborhoods are more likely to be infested than are households in neighborhoods close to the center of the city [10]. In general, the distribution of *Triatoma infestans*, the only insect vector of *T. cruzi* in the city, occurs both by active dispersal, through flying and walking, where the streets are barriers, and by passive dispersal through human movement and migration [10–12].

The collection methods have been described previously [13,14]. All insects were categorized by sex (for adults), stage, and site. A site was defined as all rooms and peri-domestic areas, such as animal enclosures, associated with a single dwelling. First instar insects did not undergo further analysis. The remaining triatomines were inspected for *T. cruzi* at the UPCH/Penn Zoonotic Disease Research Center in Arequipa, using standard techniques [15]. Briefly, we extracted feces by applying pressure to each insect's abdomen with forceps. Feces were diluted in 10 μL normal saline and examined microscopically at 400× magnification for the presence of parasites.

We built regression models to explore the relationship between *T. cruzi* prevalence and developmental stage. Due to uncertainty surrounding the total number and size of blood meals taken by adult insects, we excluded adults from our analysis. To avoid biasing our results by including a large number of insects with no potential exposure, we also excluded vectors captured at sites with no infected triatomines.

Under the Bites Hypothesis, in which the risk of acquiring the parasite is the same for each stage, the stage-prevalence relationship is given by the following cumulative binomial probability distribution:

$$P(S) = 1 - (1 - p_{bite})^S \tag{1}$$

where P is the observed infection prevalence in nymphs of stage S (i.e., $1 \leq S \leq 5$), and p_{bite} is the probability of acquiring the parasite during any given stage (Note that when $S \leq 5$ and p is sufficiently small, Equation (1) can be approximated by the linear function $P(S) \approx pS$. For example, if $p = 0.01$ and $S = 5$, then $P(S) = 0.049$ and $pS = 0.05$. This is why we hypothesized that the stage-prevalence relationship might appear roughly linear if the Bites Hypothesis were correct). To test the Bites Hypothesis, we used nonlinear least squares regression to fit Equation (1) to the observed data.

To test the Blood Hypothesis, we assumed that the risk of acquiring the parasite is the same for each milligram of blood ingested. If $B(S)$ represents the cumulative quantity (mg) of blood ingested by the average nymph of stage S, then the stage-prevalence relationship under the Blood Hypothesis is given by:

$$P(S) = 1 - (1 - p_{blood})^{B(S)} \tag{2}$$

where p_{blood} is the probability of acquiring the parasite after ingesting 1 mg of blood. The primary difference between Equations (1) and (2) is that the exponent of Equation (1) increases linearly with stage, whereas the exponent of Equation (2) increases nonlinearly. We estimated $B(S)$ from *T. infestans* feeding data in a prior study [4]. Our estimates were $B(1) = 7.1$ mg, $B(2) = 25.4$ mg, $B(3) = 87.8$ mg, $B(4) = 302.8$ mg, and $B(5) = 1072.8.0$ mg (see Appendix A for derivation). We then used nonlinear least squares regression, with $B(S)$ fixed at these values, to fit Equation (2) and estimate p_{blood} given the observed data [4].

Because the mathematical relationship between feces ingestion and infection transmission is unknown, we did not create a specific model to test the Coprophagy Hypothesis. Instead, we made a qualitative assessment of the importance of feces-mediated transmission by examining whether the other two models underestimated the infection prevalence in early-stage insects.

We used the Akaike information criterion (AIC) [16] to guide model selection. Analyses were performed in R version 3.6.3 (R Foundation for Statistical Computing, Vienna, Austria).

3. Results

We captured and analyzed 58,519 triatomines from 4138 sites. There were 188 sites (4.5%), harboring 15,252 insects, with at least one *T. cruzi*-infected triatomine. The stage distribution and *T. cruzi* prevalence of captured insects varied considerably between sites, as can be seen in Figure 2, which shows the nine infected sites with the highest number of insects. Second instars were underrepresented at most sites, possibly because it is difficult to find and capture these small nymphs. The population structure of third instars through adults was flat in some colonies (e.g., Figure 2A,C), while other colonies were skewed toward younger (Figure 2F) or older (Figure 2D) insects. These differences may be due to the age of the colonies, or they may represent heterogeneity, across sites, in stage-dependent survival. *T. cruzi* prevalence was high in some colonies (e.g., Figure 2E,I), while other colonies had only one or a few infected insects (e.g., Figure 2B–D). We speculate that the colonies with very few infected insects may represent sites where *T. cruzi* was recently introduced, perhaps via a newly infected host or migration of an infected triatomine from a nearby household. Averaged across all 188 sites, the mean prevalence of *T. cruzi* infection rose monotonically from 12% in second instars to 36% in adults (Table 1 and Figure 3).

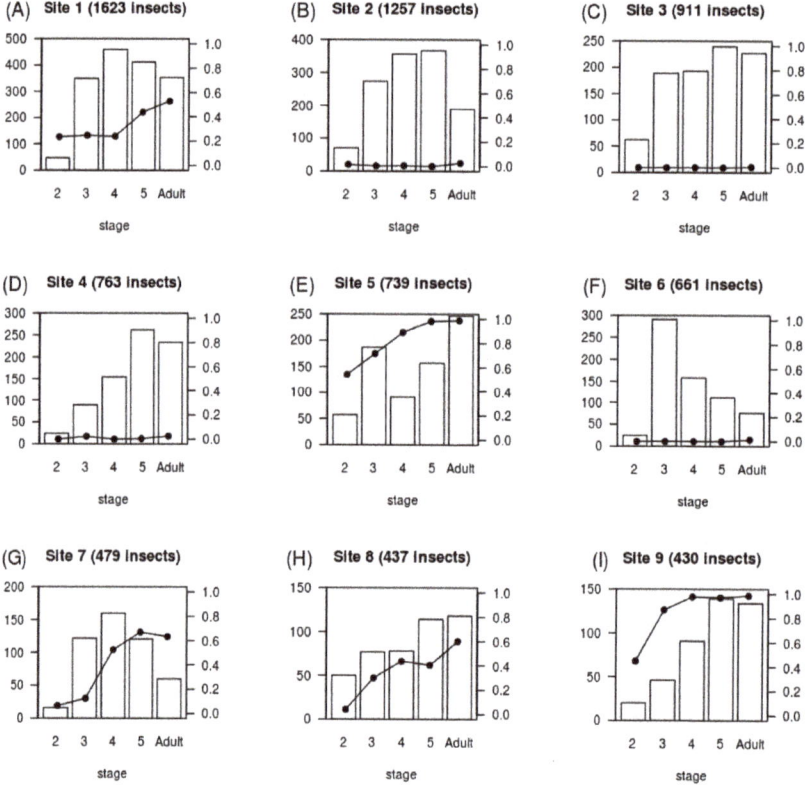

Figure 2. Distribution of developmental stage and *Trypanosoma cruzi* infection status in *Triatoma infestans* from nine households in Arequipa, Peru. Shown are the nine infected sites with the largest number of captured insects. White and black bars and left vertical axis labels: total number of insects. Black circles and right vertical axis labels: fraction of insects with *T. cruzi*.

Regression modeling demonstrated that the Bites Hypothesis was a better fit to the observations of mean *T. cruzi* prevalence versus stage (Table 2 and Figure 4). In the Bites Hypothesis model, the best-fit parameter was p_{bite} = 0.059, indicating a 5.9% probability of acquiring the parasite during any given stage. Visual inspection revealed that the Bites Hypothesis model fit the data well (Figure 4), and the model had an AIC of 11,672. In contrast, the Blood Hypothesis regression model was a very poor visual fit with a significantly higher (i.e., worse) AIC of 12,302. The observations of mean prevalence versus stage did not exhibit the excess prevalence in early nymphs that would occur if coprophagy were a primary driver of infection.

Table 1. *Trypanosoma cruzi* infection status by developmental stage, for 15,252 triatomines captured in 188 infected colonies in Arequipa, Peru.

Stage	Number Infected/Total Insects (%)
Second instar	125/1037 (12.1)
Third instar	512/3352 (15.3)
Fourth instar	687/3310 (20.8)
Fifth instar	1060/3838 (27.6)
Adult	1326/3715 (35.7)
Male	853/2225 (38.3)
Female	473/1490 (31.7)
Total	3710/15,252 (24.3)

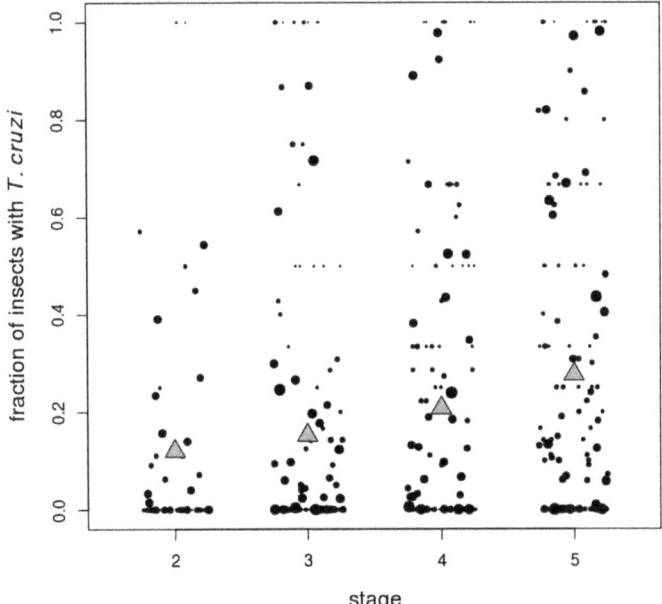

Figure 3. Fraction of nymph *Triatoma infestans* infected with *Trypanosoma cruzi* at 188 sites with at least one infected insect. Black circles represent individual sites; sizes of circles are proportional to the logarithm of the number of insects captured. The bottom edges of the gray triangles show the mean fraction of insects with *T. cruzi* across all infected sites.

Table 2. Results of regression modeling to test two hypotheses of *T. cruzi* transmission to *T. infestans*.

Model Name	Fitted Parameter	Best-Fit Parameter (95% Confidence Interval)	AIC
Bites Hypothesis	p_{bite}: probability of parasite acquisition during any given stage	p_{bite} = 0.059 (0.057 to 0.061)	11,672
Blood Hypothesis	p_{blood}: probability of parasite acquisition with each milligram of blood ingested	p_{blood} = 0.00036 (0.00035 to 0.00038)	112,302

Abbreviation: AIC, Akaike information criterion.

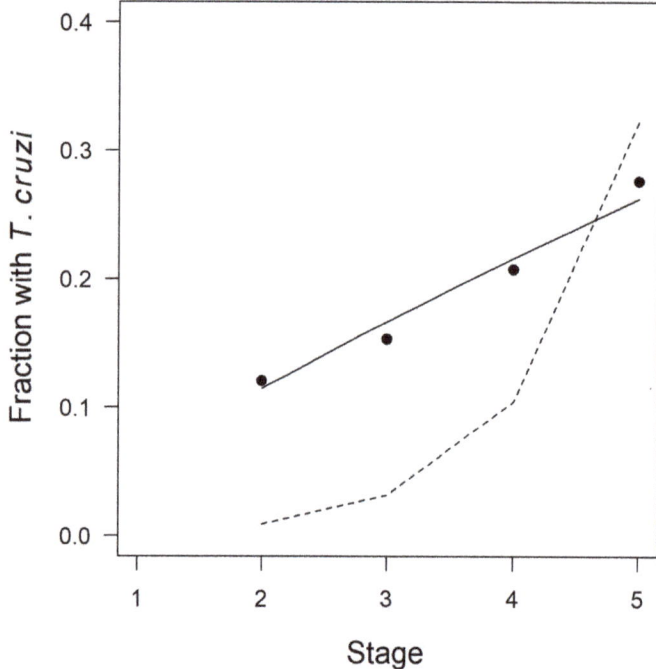

Figure 4. Fraction of triatomines infected with *Trypanosoma cruzi* as a function of stage. Filled circles: mean values observed in 15,252 insects captured at 188 infected sites. Dashed line: Best-fit regression model under the Blood Hypothesis that assumed an equal probability of infection with each milligram of blood ingested ($Pr(infection) = 1 - (1 - 0.00036)^{Nblood}$, where $Nblood$ is the number of mg of blood ingested). Solid line: Best-fit regression model under the Bites Hypothesis that assumed an equal probability of infection during any given stage ($Pr(infection) = 1 - (1 - 0.059)^N$).

4. Discussion

In a large field survey of *Triatoma infestans* captured in Arequipa, Peru, we demonstrate that the probability of *Trypanosoma cruzi* acquisition is the same at each developmental stage. This result suggests that acquisition of *T. cruzi* depends on the number of feeding opportunities (i.e., bites) and not on the quantity of blood ingested. A possible explanation for this finding is that newly infected mammalian hosts may undergo a rapid logistic increase in the number of circulating parasites. In other words, hosts may go from no parasitemia to a high level of infectiousness very quickly [17,18]. Vectors that feed on such hosts may be almost certain to acquire the parasite, regardless of the size of the blood meal they ingest. Hosts may spend only a brief amount of time at intermediate levels of parasitemia, during which time vectors acquire the parasite in proportion to the amount of blood ingested. Although this interpretation assumes that instar stage is proportional to the number of blood meals, we note that the exact relationship between these two quantities is uncertain. Some nymphs may take only one blood meal per molt, while others may take multiple blood meals per developmental stage, particularly if their feeding is interrupted before engorgement [19,20].

Our results are in general agreement with those of a prior study that reported increasing *T. cruzi* prevalence with stage in a smaller sample of wild-caught *T. infestans* nymphs and adults [21]. As in the previous study, a vector control program was ongoing in Arequipa during the time period when we collected insects. These control efforts reduced transmission of *T. cruzi* to humans [14] and decreased the population of vectors. We also confirm the results of a previous small study (n < 200) of laboratory-reared fifth instar triatomines used for xenodiagnosis, in which there was no correlation between blood meal size and the probability of *T. cruzi* infection [22].

Several reports have cast doubt on the importance of coprophagy as a route of *T. cruzi* acquisition [17,23,24]. The present study provides complementary epidemiologic evidence, from *T. infestans* captured in natural habitats, against the coprophagy route of transmission. However, since we were unable to examine first instars, more work is needed to quantify the precise role, if any, of coprophagy. It should also be noted that triatomines' need for bacterial symbionts and coprophagy have not been established with certainty. Wild-caught triatomines harbor diverse gut bacteria [6], which suggests they can acquire symbionts from routes other than coprophagy, and many triatomine species (including *T. protracta*, *T. rubida*, and *Rhodnius prolixus*) develop normally when raised in sterile environments [25].

Limitations of this study include our inability to measure the infection prevalence among first instars; our averaging of the infection prevalence across all sites, which may have oversimplified a more complex pattern of parasite transmission such as may occur in a metapopulation; and uncertainty in our assumptions regarding the number and size of blood meals consumed by triatomines of different stages. Also, the number of infected insects may have been underestimated due to the method used to detect the presence of infection in this study, which has been reported to be less sensitive than other methods such as complete insect dissection or PCR. Another limitation is that migration of infected triatomines could have biased our prevalence estimates by causing us to include colonies without well-established stable patterns of infection versus stage.

The observed pattern of *T. cruzi* prevalence versus stage could have implications for Chagas disease control strategies. Insecticides and biological control methods that preferentially kill older insects have relatively less effect on an insect's reproductive fitness and, in theory, are less likely to be rendered obsolete by evolution of resistance mechanisms [26]. Late-acting agents have been suggested as a means to combat infections including malaria [27] and Chagas disease [28]. Had we observed a highly linear increase in *T. cruzi* prevalence with stage, with few infected early-stage nymphs, we could have made a strong case for such late-acting methods. Instead, we found a substantial rate of *T. cruzi* infection in second and third instars. Although our results suggest that disproportionate killing of older triatomines may not be useful, these findings should be interpreted with caution. The probability that *T. cruzi* will be transmitted to humans depends upon several factors that we did not measure. Behavioral and physiological factors may make younger triatomines less likely to transmit the parasite. Younger instars may be less likely than adult insects to defecate on hosts [29]; may defecate longer after taking a blood meal [30]; and may be less likely to survive the parasite's incubation period, since survival of infected triatomines appears to be affected by the ratio of ingested blood to body weight [31]. Further studies will be needed to determine the relative risk of feces-mediated transmission posed by younger and older triatomines, which in turn would inform the decision of whether to pursue late-acting control strategies.

Author Contributions: Conceptualization, A.W.T., R.C.-N. and M.Z.L.; Formal analysis, A.W.T., R.C.-N. and M.Z.L.; Funding acquisition, M.Z.L.; Investigation, L.D.T., R.S. and K.B.-M.; Methodology, A.W.T. and M.Z.L.; Project administration, R.C.-N. and M.Z.L.; Supervision, R.C.-N. and M.Z.L.; Visualization, L.D.T.; Writing—original draft, A.W.T.; Writing—review and editing, L.D.T., R.C.-N. and M.Z.L. All authors have read and agreed to the published version of the manuscript.

Funding: Funding for this study came from National Institutes of Health NIAID P50 AI074285 and 5R01 AI101229.

Acknowledgments: We would like to thank the following members of the Zoonotic Disease Laboratory in Arequipa who assisted with this work: Jenny Ancca, Carlos Condori, and Jesus Pinto Caballero. We gratefully acknowledge the invaluable contributions of the Ministerio de Salud del Perú (MINSA), the Dirección General de Salud de las Personas (DGSP), the Estrategia Sanitaria Nacional de Prevención y Control de Enfermedades Metaxenicas y Otras Transmitidas por Vectores (ESNPCEMOTVS), the Dirección General de Salud Ambiental (DIGESA), the Gobierno Regional de Arequipa, la Gerencia Regional de Salud de Arequipa (GRSA), the Pan American Health Organization (PAHO/OPS), and the Canadian International Development Agency (CIDA).

Conflicts of Interest: The authors declare no conflict of interest. The funding sources had no involvement in the study design; collection, analysis, and interpretation of data; writing of the report; or decision to submit this article for publication.

Appendix A

Juarez [4] measured blood meal sizes of laboratory-reared *T. infestans* under a variety of conditions of feed source, ambient temperature, and *T. cruzi* infection status. Of the eight groups of insects studied by Juarez, the group that was uninfected, fed on chicken, and maintained at 25 °C (77 °F) was closest to the natural conditions encountered by wild insects in Arequipa. Under these conditions, Juarez found that the quantity of blood ingested during each stage increased from 7.1 mg in first instars to 770 mg in fifth instars. We used these data to estimate the cumulative quantity of blood, $B(S)$, ingested by captured wild *T. infestans* nymphs (Table A1). We assumed that insects we captured just before a molt had already ingested the stage-specific quantity of blood reported by Juarez. Under this assumption, the mean cumulative blood ingested by captured insects is simply the sum of the blood ingested during the current and all prior stages.

Table A1. Blood meal sizes observations for laboratory reared insects [4] and estimates of cumulative blood ingested by captured wild *Triatoma infestans* nymphs.

Stage	Median Quantity of Blood Ingested during this Stage (mg)	Estimated Cumulative Blood Ingested during Lifetime Prior to Capture (mg)
First instar	7.1	7.1
Second instar	18.3	25.4
Third instar	62.4	87.8
Fourth instar	215.0	302.8
Fifth instar	770.0	1072.8

References

1. Rassi, A.; Rassi, A.; Marin-Neto, J.A. Chagas disease. *Lancet* **2010**, *375*, 1388–1402. [CrossRef]
2. Schaub, G.A. Direct transmission of *Trypanosoma cruzi* between vectors of Chagas' disease. *Acta Trop.* **1988**, *45*, 11–19. [PubMed]
3. Kollien, A.H.; Schaub, G.A. The development of *Trypanosoma cruzi* (Trypanosomatidae) in the Reduviid bug *Triatoma infestans* (Insecta): Influence of starvation. *J. Eukaryot. Microbiol.* **1998**, *45*, 59–63. [CrossRef] [PubMed]
4. Juarez, E. Comportamento do *Triatoma infestans* sob várias condições de laboratório. *Rev. Saude Publica* **1970**, *4*, 147–166. [CrossRef] [PubMed]
5. Beard, C.B.; Dotson, E.M.; Pennington, P.M.; Eichler, S.; Cordon-Rosales, C.; Durvasula, R.V. Bacterial symbiosis and paratransgenic control of vector-borne Chagas disease. *Int. J. Parasitol.* **2001**, *31*, 621–627. [CrossRef]
6. Beard, C.B.; Cordon-Rosales, C.; Durvasula, R.V. Bacterial Symbionts of the Triatominae and Their Potential Use in Control of Chagas Disease Transmission. *Annu. Rev. Entomol.* **2002**, *47*, 123–141. [CrossRef]
7. Instituto Nacional de Estadística e Informática INEI. *Perú: Perfil Sociodemográfico. Censos nacionales 2017: XI de Población y VI de Vivienda*; INEI: Lima, Peru, 2018.
8. Levy, M.Z.; Barbu, C.M.; Castillo-Neyra, R.; Quispe-Machaca, V.R.; Ancca-Juarez, J.; Escalante-Mejia, P.; Borrini-Mayori, K.; Niemierko, M.; Mabud, T.S.; Behrman, J.R.; et al. Urbanization, land tenure security and vector-borne Chagas disease. *Proc. R. Soc. B Biol. Sci.* **2014**, *281*, 20141003. [CrossRef]
9. Bayer, A.M.; Hunter, G.C.; Gilman, R.H.; Cornejo Del Carpio, J.G.; Naquira, C.; Bern, C.; Levy, M.Z. Chagas disease, migration and community settlement patterns in Arequipa, Peru. *PLoS Negl. Trop. Dis.* **2009**, *3*, e567. [CrossRef]
10. Delgado, S.; Ernst, K.C.; Pumahuanca, M.L.; Yool, S.R.; Comrie, A.C.; Sterling, C.R.; Gilman, R.H.; Náquira, C.; Levy, M.Z. A country bug in the city: Urban infestation by the Chagas disease vector *Triatoma infestans* in Arequipa, Peru. *Int. J. Health Geogr.* **2013**, *12*, 48. [CrossRef]

11. Foley, E.A.; Khatchikian, C.E.; Hwang, J.; Ancca-Juárez, J.; Borrini-Mayori, K.; Quispe-Machaca, V.R.; Levy, M.Z.; Brisson, D. Population structure of the Chagas disease vector, *Triatoma infestans*, at the urban-rural interface. *Mol. Ecol.* **2013**, *22*, 5162–5171. [CrossRef]
12. Khatchikian, C.E.; Foley, E.A.; Barbu, C.M.; Hwang, J.; Ancca-Juárez, J.; Borrini-Mayori, K.; Quispe-Machaca, V.R.; Naquira, C.; Brisson, D.; Levy, M.Z. Population Structure of the Chagas Disease Vector *Triatoma infestans* in an Urban Environment. *PLoS Negl. Trop. Dis.* **2015**, *9*, e0003425. [CrossRef] [PubMed]
13. Levy, M.Z.; Bowman, N.M.; Kawai, V.; Waller, L.A.; Del Carpio, J.G.C.; Benzaquen, E.C.; Gilman, R.H.; Bern, C. Periurban *Trypanosoma cruzi*-infected *Triatoma infestans*, Arequipa, Peru. *Emerg. Infect. Dis.* **2006**, *12*, 1345–1352. [CrossRef] [PubMed]
14. Delgado, S.; Castillo Neyra, R.; Quispe Machaca, V.R.; Ancca Juárez, J.; Chou Chu, L.; Verastegui, M.R.; Moscoso Apaza, G.M.; Bocángel, C.D.; Tustin, A.W.; Sterling, C.R.; et al. A history of chagas disease transmission, control, and re-emergence in peri-rural La Joya, Peru. *PLoS Negl. Trop. Dis.* **2011**, *5*, e970. [CrossRef] [PubMed]
15. Gurtler, R.E.; Cohen, J.E.; Cecere, M.C.; Lauricella, M.A.; Chuit, R.; Segura, E.L. Influence of humans and domestic animals on the household prevalence of *Trypanosoma cruzi* in *Triatoma infestans* populations in northwest Argentina. *Am. J. Trop. Med. Hyg.* **1998**, *58*, 748–758. [CrossRef]
16. Akaike, H. A new look at the statistical model identification. *IEEE Trans. Automat. Contr.* **1974**, *19*, 716–723. [CrossRef]
17. Levy, M.Z.; Tustin, A.; Castillo-Neyra, R.; Mabud, T.S.; Levy, K.; Barbu, C.M.; Quispe-Machaca, V.R.; Ancca-Juarez, J.; Borrini-Mayori, K.; Naquira-Velarde, C.; et al. Bottlenecks in domestic animal populations can facilitate the emergence of *Trypanosoma cruzi*, the aetiological agent of Chagas disease. *Proc. R. Soc. B Biol. Sci.* **2015**, *282*, 20142807. [CrossRef]
18. Castillo-Neyra, R.; Borrini Mayorí, K.; Salazar Sánchez, R.; Ancca Suarez, J.; Xie, S.; Náquira Velarde, C.; Levy, M.Z. Heterogeneous infectiousness in guinea pigs experimentally infected with *Trypanosoma cruzi*. *Parasitol. Int.* **2016**, *65*, 50–54. [CrossRef]
19. Gürtler, R.E.; Ceballos, L.A.; Ordóñez-Krasnowski, P.; Lanati, L.A.; Stariolo, R.; Kitron, U. Strong host-feeding preferences of the vector *Triatoma infestans* modified by vector density: Implications for the epidemiology of Chagas disease. *PLoS Negl. Trop. Dis.* **2009**, *3*, e447. [CrossRef]
20. Catalá, S.S.; Noireau, F.; Dujardin, J.-P. Biology of Triatominae. In *American Trypanosomiasis Chagas Disease*; Elsevier: Amsterdam, The Netherlands, 2017; pp. 145–167.
21. Cecere, M.C.; Castañera, M.B.; Canale, D.M.; Chuit, R.; Gürtler, R.E. *Trypanosoma cruzi* infection in *Triatoma infestans* and other triatomines: Long-term effects of a control program in rural northwestern Argentina. *Rev. Panam. Salud Pública* **1999**, *5*, 392–399. [CrossRef]
22. Miles, M.A.; Patterson, J.W.; Marsden, P.D.; Minter, D.M. A comparison of *Rhodnius prolixus*, *Triatoma infestans* and *Panstrongylus megistus* in the xenodiagnosis of a chronic *Trypanosoma* (Schizotrypanum) *cruzi* infection in a rhesus monkey (*Macaca mullatta*). *Trans. R. Soc. Trop. Med. Hyg.* **1975**, *69*, 377–382. [CrossRef]
23. Torres, M. Alguns fatos que interessam á epidemiolojia da molestia de Chagas. *Mem. Inst. Oswaldo Cruz* **1915**, *7*, 120–138.
24. Phillips, N.R. Experimental Studies on the Quantitative Transmission of *Trypanosoma Cruzi*: Aspects of the Rearing, Maintenance and Testing of Vector Material, and of the Origin and Course of Infection in the Vector. *Ann. Trop. Med. Parasitol.* **1960**, *54*, 397–414. [CrossRef] [PubMed]
25. Nyirady, S.A. The Germfree Culture of Three Species of Triatominae: *Triatoma Protracta* (Uhler), *Triatoma Rubida* (Uhler) and *Rhodnius Prolixus* StÅL1. *J. Med. Entomol.* **1973**, *10*, 417–448. [CrossRef] [PubMed]
26. Read, A.F.; Lynch, P.A.; Thomas, M.B. How to make evolution-proof insecticides for malaria control. *PLoS Biol.* **2009**, *7*, 0001–00010. [CrossRef]
27. Koella, J.C.; Lynch, P.A.; Thomas, M.B.; Read, A.F. Towards evolution-proof malaria control with insecticides. *Evol. Appl.* **2009**, *2*, 469–480. [CrossRef]
28. Forlani, L.; Pedrini, N.; Girotti, J.R.; Mijailovsky, S.J.; Cardozo, R.M.; Gentile, A.G.; Hernández-Suárez, C.M.; Rabinovich, J.E.; Juárez, M.P. Biological Control of the Chagas Disease Vector *Triatoma infestans* with the Entomopathogenic Fungus Beauveria bassiana Combined with an Aggregation Cue: Field, Laboratory and Mathematical Modeling Assessment. *PLoS Negl. Trop. Dis.* **2015**, *9*, 1–23. [CrossRef]

29. Dias, E. Observações sôbre eliminação de dejeções e tempo de sucção em alguns triatomíneos sul-americanos. *Mem. Inst. Oswaldo Cruz* **1956**, *54*, 115–124. [CrossRef]
30. Trumper, E.V.; Gorla, D.E. Density-dependent timing of defaecation by *Triatoma infestans*. *Trans. R. Soc. Trop. Med. Hyg.* **1991**, *85*, 800–802. [CrossRef]
31. Peterson, J.K.; Graham, A.L.; Dobson, A.P.; Chávez, O.T. *Rhodnius prolixus* life history outcomes differ when infected with different *trypanosoma cruzi* i strains. *Am. J. Trop. Med. Hyg.* **2015**, *93*, 564–572. [CrossRef]

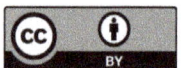 © 2020 by the authors. Licensee MDPI, Basel, Switzerland. This article is an open access article distributed under the terms and conditions of the Creative Commons Attribution (CC BY) license (http://creativecommons.org/licenses/by/4.0/).

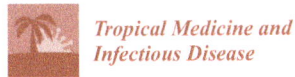

Article

Chagas Disease and Healthcare Rights in the Bolivian Immigrant Community of São Paulo, Brazil

Fernando Mussa Abujamra Aith [1,*], Colin Forsyth [2] and Maria Aparecida Shikanai-Yasuda [3,*]

1. Department of Preventive Medicine, Faculdade de Medicina, University of São Paulo, Av. Dr. Arnaldo, 455. Cerqueira César; São Paulo, SP 01246-903, Brazil
2. Drugs for Neglected Diseases initiative, Rua São José 70 #601, Centro. Rio de Janeiro, RJ 20010-020, Brazil; cforsyth@dndi.org
3. Department of Infectious Diseases, Faculdade de Medicina, University of São Paulo, Av. Dr. Arnaldo, 455. Cerqueira César; São Paulo, SP 01246-903, Brazil
* Correspondence: fernando.aith@usp.br (F.M.A.A.); masyasuda@yahoo.com.br (M.A.S.-Y.)

Received: 13 February 2020; Accepted: 14 April 2020; Published: 17 April 2020

Abstract: Chagas disease (CD) poses a major public health challenge for the Americas and non endemic regions around the world. This study discusses the legal framework surrounding access to healthcare for CD for Bolivian migrants living in São Paulo, Brazil. While recent guidelines stipulating care for CD exist, there is a lack of legal provisions to ensure they are regularly implemented. Bolivian migrants in SP have specific needs, including language differences and a high level of mobility. Interviews were conducted with ten participants representing public health institutions or organizations working with the Bolivian migrant community. Additionally, a review was conducted of legal, official, and health policy documents pertaining to rights of Bolivian migrants in SP. Although the right to healthcare is constitutionally guaranteed for all, in practice, immigrants, especially those without documentation, encounter barriers to initiating treatment for CD. Providing the primary health care system (SUS) card would not only improve access to healthcare for Bolivian migrants, but also provide a potential pathway toward regularization of status. The approval of clinical protocols and therapeutic guidelines for CD (2018) represents an opportunity to improve care for all Brazilians with CD. Programs with multidisciplinary teams should be developed taking into account the specific social and cultural needs of this population.

Keywords: Chagas disease; neglected tropical diseases; migration; healthcare rights

1. Background

Over six million people are infected with *Trypanosoma cruzi*, the parasite that causes Chagas disease (CD) [1–3]. Like other neglected tropical diseases (NTDs), CD is concentrated among poor, marginalized populations with limited access to healthcare. Moreover, there are substantial gaps in both research and development and public health infrastructure; effective new drugs for CD have not been developed in nearly 50 years, and less than one percent of people with the infection have received diagnosis and treatment in the Americas [4–6]. This leads to a considerable burden of morbidity and mortality, since, in the absence of timely identification and treatment, CD leads to serious, life-threatening complications (most often heart disease) in 30%–40% of those infected with *T. cruzi*. These complications most frequently manifest in individuals who are at the peak of their productive years (30–50 years old), creating immense voids in families and communities [7,8]. Brazil, where CD was originally discovered by Carlos Chagas in 1909, has the second-largest burden of the disease worldwide, with over 1.1 million people infected, and incurs the highest annual healthcare costs from CD, estimated at $129 million in 2013 (equivalent to $143 million in 2020) [1,9].

CD's epidemiological profile has transformed in recent decades [10]. In the twentieth century, CD was principally confined to rural areas of Latin America. However, at the millennium's close, political violence and economic necessity fueled rural–urban migration within Latin America as well as international migration to Europe, North America, and Asia [10,11]. Migrants in these new settings face significant political, economic, and sociocultural challenges to accessing healthcare for CD [12–15].

São Paulo, the world's fifth largest city [16] and a major destination for immigrants from across the globe, illustrates the changing epidemiology of CD. Annual immigration to Brazil increased from 143,600 in 2000 to 268,400 a decade later [16]. Bolivia stands out as the fifth country with the highest flow of immigration to Brazil, and the city of São Paulo (SP) is the most common destination for Bolivian migrants. In effect, although the presence of Bolivian immigrants in the border areas of Mato Grosso do Sul, Mato Grosso, Rondônia, and Acre is significant, there is a high concentration of Bolivian immigrants in the metropolitan region of São Paulo.

Estimates indicate there are over 350,000 Bolivians living in SP [17]; 44.1% work in the garment industry, while others work as street vendors, doctors, and dentists [16,18]. The majority of Bolivian immigrants in São Paulo are men, who have been living in the country for more than 10 years. When arriving to São Paulo, Bolivian migrants confront a new reality of life, full of cultural, linguistic, and social differences. This situation places them in a condition of physical, psychological, and social vulnerability, which can directly influence their health status [16,19]. This vulnerability is further compounded for people who lack required documentation [20].

Bolivia, where over 600,000 people are infected with *T. cruzi*, has the highest global CD prevalence (6.1%) [1]. CD is also a major concern for Bolivian migrants living in SP. A recent study found a seroprevalence of 4.4% in this population [21]. Other major global cities where migrants face healthcare access challenges for CD include Los Angeles [22], Munich [23], Rome [24], London [25], Buenos Aires [26], and Barcelona [27].

Brazil has a long history of public health efforts devoted to CD, and domiciliary vector transmission in SP state was interrupted in the 1960s. Nevertheless, access to etiological treatment for CD via the primary healthcare system (Unified Health System, Sistema Único de Saúde, or SUS) remains a significant challenge, not only for large numbers of Brazilians who have migrated to SP from endemic areas, but for Bolivian migrants, who present unique social, political, legal, and cultural needs, and represent a new reality for SP's healthcare system in terms of demand for health services, morbidity, and vulnerability.

The World Health Organization has made the right to health a fundamental pillar of its global strategy to combat neglected tropical diseases, while universal health coverage is considered essential to achieving the United Nations Sustainable Development Goals [28]. Nonetheless, gains in extending health coverage to vulnerable groups, especially immigrants, are in jeopardy from the rise of far-right, authoritarian-leaning governments across the globe, a phenomenon that has recently impacted Brazil. This article identifies the extent of migrants' right to health in Brazil, and analyzes how this impacts utilization of the SUS and other public services for CD management. This work aims at improving understanding of migrants' therapeutic itinerary for CD. The research was conducted as part of a larger study on the socioepidemiological and clinical characteristics of CD and access to healthcare among Bolivian migrants in SP [21,29,30].

2. Methods

Two types of primary data were used for this study: interviews of key respondents and relevant legal, technical, and policy documents.

2.1. Participants

Ten semistructured interviews (see semistructured interview script in the supplementary file) were conducted with respondents from the following institutions: The Secretaries of Health of the State and Municipality of SP; Bolivia's Consul in SP; the Federal Prosecutor and Public Defender;

Pastoral Migrants Service in SP, the Association of Bolivian Residents (ADRB), and the Kantuta Bolivian Association.

2.2. Data Collection

Interviews focused on Bolivian migrants' health rights were conducted in 2014 and 2015 by a researcher with expertise on human rights and public health issues. The interviews followed a semistructured guide (annex) with 10 questions about respondents' activities, particularly regarding migrants, and opinions/perspectives regarding the Bolivian community in São Paulo. Participants were selected based on their professional background and strategic position in institutions with public or official activities and programs related to Bolivian migration and the health system. Content analysis of the interviews suggested that the method reached saturation once data collection began to be repetitive. The interviews were recorded after obtaining consent from participants. Interviews were transcribed as Word documents, then analyzed and coded for themes related to interviewees' activities, opinions, and perspectives related to the health care for migrants in SP, as well as suggestions of key documentation and references.

In addition to the interviews, we conducted a review of official legal and technical documents. From March 2014 to March 2016, we reviewed legislative and normative guidelines pertaining to the legal status of Bolivian immigrants in Brazil, as well as their health rights and possibilities to freely access Brazilian public health services, especially as pertains to CD. The review included only official government websites and legislative data from the Federal Government (www.planalto.gov.br), the Ministry of Health (http://portal2.saude.gov.br/saudelegis and http://portalms.saude.gov.br/protocolos-e-diretrizes), the Health Secretariat of the State of SP (www.saude.sp.gov.br), and the Health Secretariat of the Municipality of SP (MSP) (http://www.prefeitura.sp.gov.br/cidade/secretarias/saude/). Special attention was given to the current legal and normative technical documents that organize and structure the Brazilian public health system at the national, regional, and local levels, and to specific public policies regarding immigrants and CD.

For the documents search, key words were immigrants, immigration, Chagas disease, Clinical Protocols, Clinical Guidelines, right to health, and health rights. Our search resulted in 141 records; 62 legal and normative documents related to immigrants and 79 clinical protocols and guidelines approved by the Ministry of Health. We reviewed each record and only retained legal and normative documents related to immigration status, public policies on CD, or health surveillance ($n = 12$).

The Research Ethics Committee of the Clinical Hospital of the School of Medicine, University of SP approved the research, and the interviewees signed the respective Terms of Free and Informed Consent.

3. Results

The healthcare rights of Bolivians with CD living in SP depend on three important frameworks: (1) their legal status in Brazil, particularly as it pertains to accessing healthcare via the SUS; (2) policies and legal requirements regarding provision of testing and treatment for CD; and (3) capacity of the health system to provide care for Bolivians with CD.

3.1. Legal Status Considerations for Bolivian Migrants in SP

The legal and normative documents related to immigrants, collected during the research provided insight on how Brazilian legislation treats Bolivian immigrants regarding the right to health.

Brazilian Law 6.815/1980 (known as the Foreigners' Statute) [31] indicates visas may be granted to foreign nationals who enter Brazil and meet certain legal requirements. Article Five of the Federal Constitution affirms that foreign nationals living in Brazil enjoy the same legal status and rights as Brazilians. However, whenever required by any authority or agent, foreigners must show official documentation attesting to their legal permission to reside in Brazil. In cases of irregular entry or unauthorized residence of a foreign national in Brazilian territory, authorities will first demand voluntary removal, and failing this, will initiate deportation procedures.

Obtaining the necessary documents to remain in Brazil poses a significant challenge, putting at risk migrants' right to access healthcare. First, to obtain official residence in Brazil, a migrant must first produce original personal documents from their country of origin. These documents can sometimes only be obtained through the Bolivian Consulate. After that, a series of bureaucratic processes including forms and payments must be completed through the Brazilian Federal Police Department. This includes going in person to the local police office. These cumbersome and potentially intimidating processes can make it very difficult for migrants to regularize their status. According to one respondent from an NGO working with Bolivian migrants, "there are some bureaucratic obstacles in the Brazilian and Bolivian governments that make it difficult to obtain documents, and this ends up having repercussions on the enjoyment of rights".

Brazil's Migration Amnesty Law [32] provides an opportunity for undocumented migrants who had entered the country prior to February 1, 2009, to regularize their status and obtain freedom of movement, the right to work, and access to public services, including healthcare. While this represented a potentially strong advance in the protection of the rights of Bolivian and other immigrants, interviewees report that a lack of documentation continues to be a major concern. The Bolivian General Consul estimates there are around 50,000 Bolivians in SP in need of regularizing their status, and not having proper documentation represents a major barrier to accessing public health services. Interviewees indicated Bolivian immigrants often feel strong apprehension or fear that attempts to access healthcare will expose their status, subjecting them to repercussions including fines and deportation. As reported by one Bolivian migrant representative, "if I give my address and this kind of information in the hospital, not being legal in the country, they will go after me as soon as they realize I do not have the proper visa to be in Brazil and they will want to send me back". One of the public officials interviewed confirmed this reality: "Migrants without proper documents can legally be submitted to some enforcement measures such as arrest or deportation".

Thus, although immigrants' access to healthcare is guaranteed as a constitutional right, this is in large part negated by the difficulty of obtaining the documentation needed to secure legal residency. As reported by a public official responsible for immigration issues, "sometimes the migrant comes to us to ask for a kind of document assuring that they have the right to be treated in SUS facilities even if they do not have legal status in the Country ... ; and they come to us because they have already tried to be treated and the public service denied access because they do not have the proper documents to show". It is important to state that migrants in Brazil, even undocumented, have the constitutional right to access public health services (even if they do not show any identity document and proof of residence). In these cases, they can go to public defenders or to the Public Ministry to ask for a document able to protect their right to health. Although this documentation can improve access from a legal standpoint, other linguistic, sociocultural, and CD-specific healthcare barriers, remain.

3.2. Legal Status and Healthcare Access

According to articles 5 and 196 of the Brazilian Constitution, the access of Bolivian migrants to public health services must occur in the same way as for Brazilian citizens. Migrants in Brazil, regardless of status, have the same health rights as Brazilians, including access to health services and treatments. Table 1 outlines the major portals of entry by which Brazilians or Bolivians living in SP might enter the SUS [33] as defined by governmental laws, which standardize the entry process. Whenever a new patient enters through one of these doors, they will receive a SUS card, entitling the recipient to: primary care services from Family Health Strategy facilities; office visits for primary care services, including vaccinations; home visits conducted by the Family Health Strategy; emergency care; and mental health services [34].

The Family Health Strategy (FHS) seeks to promote the quality of life of the Brazilian population and address factors that put health at risk, such as lack of physical activity, poor diet, and the use of tobacco. With comprehensive, equitable, and continuous care, the FHS serves as a gateway to the public Unified Health System (SUS) in Brazil. The FHS is composed of a multidisciplinary team that has at least one general practitioner or family health doctor, one nursing assistant, two nursing technicians and several community health agents (CHAs) to cover 100% of the registered population with a maximum of 750 people per agent and 12 CHAs per Family Health team [34]. There can also be an oral health team, consisting of a general dentist and a technician in oral health. Each Family Health team is responsible for a maximum of 4000 people from a given area [34].

Table 1. Entry points to the Unified Health System (Sistema Único de Saúd—SUS) for Bolivian immigrants in the city of São Paulo, Brazil.

SUS Entry Points	Health Services
Primary Healthcare Facilities	• Outpatient care • Laboratory tests • Pharmacies • Vaccination programs • Other basic health services
Family Health Strategy (FHS)	• Home visits by FHS teams • In-person care at SUS clinics generated by FHS home visits
Emergency Units	• Emergency services (emergency room)
Center for Psychosocial Care	• Mental health services

Many facilities within the health system will provide the card needed to utilize SUS healthcare services regardless of documentation status. In fact, all interviewees reported the SUS card was often the first official Brazilian document obtained by Bolivian migrants from a public authority, emphasizing that access to the health system may represent the first contact with the State and a potential starting point for status regularization. Within the SUS, there is no regulation stipulating that foreigners receive different types of care than Brazilian nationals. Municipal and state health authorities in SP also indicate that there is no specific therapeutic protocol pertaining to care for immigrants.

3.3. Legal and Policy Framework for CD Healthcare

In 2011, Brazilian Law 12.401 mandated the creation of official clinical protocols and therapeutic guidelines for specific diseases [33]. While Brazilian experts had published two consensus documents on CD [8], the Ministry of Health had not put forth a clinical protocol for CD during the period of data collection. Aside from the consensus documents, there were basic manuals of care for CD [35], and regional guidelines for care of CD cardiomyopathy [36] and oral CD [37], but there were no legal provisions to enforce the recommendations in these documents. However, on 30 October, 2018, a clinical protocol for diagnosis and therapeutic guidelines (Protocolo Clinico de Diretrizes Terapeuticas, PCDT) for CD was approved by the National Commission for Incorporation of Technology into the SUS (Comissão Nacional de Incorporação de Tecnologias no SUS, or CONITEC) [38]. The PCDT contained several provisions to strengthen access to healthcare for people with CD, including obligatory reporting of chronic cases, measures to reinforce referral pathways and provision of etiological treatment at the primary level, and strengthening of recommendations to etiologically treat chronically infected adults up to age 50, especially women of childbearing age. The PCDT does not contain special provisions for migrants in the main document, so its recommendations are valid for all individuals registered in the SUS. However, the tone of the PCDT's supporting annexes suggests that routine treatment would not be recommended for migrants, based on a lower rate of PCR conversion after antiparasitic treatment in Argentina, Bolivia, and Colombia compared to Brazil [39]. As this data is based on the analysis of only one study population, whereas other observational studies in different contexts do suggest clinical benefits from antiparasitic treatment in various populations [40–44], it deserves further discussion, lest this provision impede the ability of migrants to enjoy the right to healthcare in the form of antiparasitic treatment.

3.4. Needs within the Health System

Interviews revealed several challenges within the health system regarding provision of care for CD to Bolivian migrants. Table 2 displays the challenges highlighted by the interviewees, identifying the major gaps and related outcomes.

4. Discussion

Requiring documentation poses a major deterrent for Bolivian immigrants who do not enjoy regular status, as Brazilian health facilities require one document of identification and one proof of residence in the city to proceed with treatment. This protocol can be more flexible when the Family Health Team visits the patient, since in these cases proof of residence is not required. Additionally, the different epidemiological profile of the disease in Bolivia could create different clinical issues; for example, women who have resided in endemic areas may have a greater risk of transmitting CD to their infants in utero. In fact, prior research found a 6.1% prevalence of *T. cruzi* infection in Bolivian women of reproductive age living in São Paulo [21], substantially higher than reported prevalence among Brazilian women in endemic areas (1.1%) [45]. Moreover, some clinical parameters including morbidity may differ between people infected in Bolivia or Brazil, as reported [29], largely due to the younger age of the Bolivian migrant population with CD. Interviewees also stressed provider–patient language differences as an important barrier, rendering it difficult for patients to understand explanations of their diagnosis or instructions for treatment. In addition, like other migrant populations, Bolivians with CD are highly mobile, which can make long-term follow-up challenging. Mobility from São Paulo to Bolivia or from one district to another in the city of São Paulo has contributed to a high rate (42.1%) of abandonment of antiparasitic treatment [29].

One of the main gaps revealed in our research was the lack of a specific therapeutic protocol (PCDT) for CD, despite the stipulation in favor of creating such a protocol by Brazilian Law 12.401 in 2011. The approval of the PCDT for CD in October, 2018 [38], presents an opportunity to increase access to care for CD for all affected people in Brazil. However, neither the PCDT, nor the prior legal framework, contain special provisions relating to the care of migrants. Respondents indicated that there are no provisions or programs in place to ensure migrants from known endemic areas receive timely diagnosis and care.

As the results illustrate, another important gap is related to the right of immigrants to obtain healthcare on an equal footing with Brazilian citizens, as affirmed by Brazil's Constitution. In practice the requirement for producing documentation in order to receive services poses a key barrier, even considering that this is not a uniform practice. Some providers related to Family Health Teams do not require documentation prior to seeing patients, whereas others, related to Health Facilities, turn away undocumented patients.

In different countries and health systems, migrants with CD have faced key challenges to accessing care and often represent a particularly vulnerable group. In the United States and Europe, for example, immigration status can pose a major barrier to obtaining care for people with CD [12,14,46,47]. In Brazil, bureaucratic processes to obtain legal documents are potentially intimidating and make it very difficult for migrants to regularize their status.

Table 2. Gaps in care of Bolivian immigrants with Chagas disease in São Paulo's public health system.

GAPS	Description in the Interviews	Outcomes
1. Requiring documentation discourages patients from utilizing primary healthcare services.	"We know of those who are registered, but we know that there are many who do not have documents" (Interviewee* 1). "In relation to foreigners, we have a problem with the SUS card. Many foreigners have difficulty understanding the SUS system, understanding how they have access." (Interviewee* 2).	• Missed opportunity to provide timely treatment and reduce morbidity/mortality. • Missed opportunity to halt vertical transmission Non-attendance.
2. Unitary approach to healthcare for Chagas disease.	"There is a large concentration of migrants, but they do not go to the doctor. Because they are mistreated, they do not go (…)" (Interviewee* 3).	• Failure to address different needs in terms of morbidity according to the country of origin.
3. Language differences. Lack of professionals able to communicate in languages other than Portuguese.	"The main one would be regarding language, healthcare services in Brazil are poorly paid, people are stressed, they are poorly paid, someone who does not know the language arrives and is already mistreated" (Interviewee* 3). "Firstly, we identify where our Bolivian patient is located with our teams, so we have already seen that there is a problem with the language filling in the forms, so the materials produced are now also being made in Spanish." (Interviewee* 4). "They complain a lot about prejudice, but I think that the biggest problem is that of language, which generates ill will among public workers who serve them". (Interviewee* 5).	• Non-comprehension of the diagnosis or the therapy to be followed. • Lower intention to search for the health service. • Decreased adherence to the treatment.
4. Movement of immigrants within and beyond the city.	"Immigrants are spread over the Administrative Districts: Brás, Sé, Vila Maria and Vila Guilherme, mainly" (Interviewee* 6). "First, we know that they are located in the last two decades, in the region of the East Zone, Center, more towards the East Zone, Mooca, Brás, go to Penha, Guarulhos, there is a concentration there. (…). And also, without a doubt, we have those inside. In Carapicuíba we also have, a little in Osasco, we even have Americana already. And Guarulhos without a doubt, and all continuity in São Paulo. Penha, from where Guarulhos continues, we have a large concentration of Bolivians who are working here on sewing" (Interviewee* 7).	• Incorrect or outdated addresses and contact information. • Greater challenges adhering to long-term treatment regimens.
5. Lack of reference and counter-reference health services for patients diagnosed with CD.	"Routine examinations are not yet carried out on Chagas disease, but there is already a discussion on the problem and guidance to obstetricians and gynecologists to request the examination in adults with epidemiological history and pregnant women". (Interviewee* 6). "To my knowledge, there is no reference and counter-reference network. A network does not exist. Some individual initiatives have … . If there is a group developing some research, it opens an outpatient clinic to assist the patient. It is the units that are the school centers, right? For research." (Interviewee* 4).	• Lack of specific guidelines within the public health system for the management of CD patients. • Lack of prior case histories and other clinical information for patients who are diagnosed with CD, or for previously diagnosed patients who need to see specialists due to complications.

• *Interviewee* 1: Representative of the Migrants Pastoral Service in SP; Interviewee* 2: Representative of Federal Public Defender Office; Interviewee* 3: Representative of Bolivians Association of Kantuta (São Paulo City); Interviewee* 4: Primary Care Center Director on São Paulo City, Interviewee* 5: Representative the Human Rights Committee of the São Paulo City Parliament; Interviewee* 6: Basic Care Coordinator of São Paulo City, Interviewee* 7: Representative of Bolivia's Consulate São Paulo, Brazil.

Moreover, CD has persistently remained a neglected disease despite the existence of universal health coverage in endemic [6] as well as nonendemic countries [46]. In addition to legal barrier and gaps in healthcare systems, migrants with CD must navigate linguistic and cultural differences with healthcare personnel. People diagnosed with CD may experience fear regarding the implications of the disease and stigma because of its association with poverty and rurality [13].

It is worth highlighting that the health system of the MSP has the capacity to treat CD in both immigrants and Brazilians. There is, therefore, the practical possibility of creating well-defined therapeutic itineraries for CD in SP and, thereby reducing the risks of aggravation of this disease in diagnosed patients. We propose positioning the public health system as a port of entry to guarantee immigrants' right to health, and other rights, through the Family Health Strategy [34]. Through this channel, the SUS card could be provided, not only assuring better access to health services but, in many cases, also providing the first official document in Brazil, facilitating a pathway toward regularization of status. Ideally, coverage through the Family Health Strategy in the city of São Paulo will allow teams to identify the immigrant population and their health needs, strengthening the health relationship with this group.

Significant improvements in access to treatment for CD for the Bolivian community will depend on collaboration and dialogue between health services; municipal, state, and federal authorities; the Bolivian Consulate, and organizations working within SP's Bolivian community. Special programs that take into account the sociocultural needs of the Bolivian community are needed, and such programs should include training of local healthcare personnel to improve interactions with Bolivian patients.

In the interest of promoting an open society supporting those seeking better lives and working conditions, the Federal Constitution assures immigrants the same rights as Brazilian citizens, and also guarantees healthcare as a human right [48]. The management/treatment of Bolivian immigrants by the SUS is therefore a duty of the state and society. A legal framework exists supporting the right of Bolivian migrants to obtain healthcare for CD, which could potentially produce an important reduction in morbimortality and an improvement in quality of life. However, important challenges remain before Brazil's immigrant community can freely exercise their right to treatment for CD and other diseases.

Finally, a key limitation of this work is the low number of interviewees, although data analyses suggested that the saturation level was reached since some information became repetitive. This is possibly explained because the invited responders are in strategic positions concerning health care access in the city of São Paulo. Nonetheless, further ethnographic research with people affected by CD in São Paulo, as well as workers within the health system, could illuminate other important aspects of migrants' access to health.

5. Declarations

Ethical Approval: The Research Ethics Committee of the Clinical Hospital of the School of Medicine, University of São Paulo approved the research (N°. 196.698/2013).

Consent for Publication: Not applicable.

Availability of Data and Materials: The datasets used and/or analyzed during the current study are available from the corresponding author on reasonable request.

Supplementary Materials: The following are available online at http://www.mdpi.com/2414-6366/5/2/62/s1, Semi-structured interview script.

Author Contributions: F.M.A.A. designed the study, participated in project administration, collected and analyzed data, wrote/reviewed the manuscript, and prepared the tables. C.F. wrote/reviewed the manuscript and prepared the tables. M.A.S.-Y. designed the study: wrote/reviewed the manuscript, responsible for funding acquisition and project administrations. All authors have read and agreed to the published version of the manuscript.

Funding: Financial support was provided by the Brazilian National Council for Scientific and Technological Development: 404336/2012-4. The funder was not involved in study design; collection, analysis, and interpretation of data; or writing the manuscript.

Acknowledgments: We would like to thank the Chagas Disease: Basic Care and Immigration Research Group (Nivaldo Carneiro Jr, Expedito Luna, Dalva M. V. Wanderley, Rubens A. Silva, Cássio Silveira, Lia M. Brito Silva, Noemia Barbosa Carvalho, Magda Atala, Rosário Q. Ferrufino, Luzia Martinelli, Camila Sáfolo, and Sonia Regina de Almeida). DNDi is grateful to its donors, public and private, who have provided funding to DNDi since its inception in 2003. A full list of DNDi donors can be found at http://www.dndi.org/donors/donors.

Conflicts of Interest: The authors declare no conflict of interest.

References

1. World Health Organization. Chagas disease in Latin America: An epidemiological update based on 2010 estimates. *Wkly Epidemiol Rec.* **2015**, *6*, 7.
2. Manne-Goehler, J.; Umeh, C.A.; Montgomery, S.P.; Wirtz, V.J. Estimating the Burden of Chagas Disease in the United States. *PLoS Negl. Trop. Dis.* **2016**, *10*, e0005033. [CrossRef] [PubMed]
3. Basile, L.; Jansa, J.M.; Carlier, Y.; Salamanca, D.D.; Angheben, A.; Bartoloni, A.; Seixas, J.; Van Gool, T.; Cañavate, C.; Flores-Chávez, M.; et al. Chagas disease in European countries: The challenge of a surveillance system. Euro surveillance Bulletin Europeen sur les maladies transmissibles. *Europ. Commun. Dis. Bull.* **2011**, *16*, 19968.
4. Manne, J.M.; Snively, C.S.; Ramsey, J.M.; Salgado, M.O.; Barnighausen, T.; Reich, M.R. Barriers to treatment access for Chagas disease in Mexico. *PLoS Negl. Trop. Dis.* **2013**, *7*, e2488. [CrossRef]
5. Manne-Goehler, J.; Reich, M.R.; Wirtz, V.J. Access to Care for Chagas Disease in the United States: A Health Systems Analysis. *Am. J. Trop. Med. Hyg.* **2015**, *93*, 108–113. [CrossRef]
6. Cucunubá, Z.M.; Manne-Goehler, J.M.; Díaz, D.; Nouvellet, P.; Bernal, O.; Marchiol, A.; Basáñez, M.G.; Conteh, L. How universal is coverage and access to diagnosis and treatment for Chagas disease in Colombia? A health systems analysis. *Soc. Sci. Med.* **2017**, *175*, 187–198. [CrossRef]
7. Rassi, A., Jr.; Rassi, S.G.; Rassi, A. Sudden death in Chagas' disease. *Arq. Bras Cardiol.* **2001**, *76*, 75–96. [CrossRef]
8. Dias, J.C.P.; Ramos, A.N., Jr.; Gontijo, E.D.; Luquetti, A.; Shikanai-Yasuda, M.A.; Coura, J.R.; Torres, R.M.; Melo, J.R.D.C.; Almeida, E.A.D.; Oliveira, W.D., Jr.; et al. Second Brazilian Consensus on Chagas Disease. *Rev. Soc. Bras. Med. Trop.* **2016**, *49*, 3–60. [CrossRef]
9. Lee, B.Y.; Bacon, K.M.; Bottazzi, M.E.; Hotez, P.J. Global economic burden of Chagas disease: A computational simulation model. *Lancet Infect. Dis.* **2013**, *13*, 342–348. [CrossRef]
10. Briceno-Leon, R. Chagas disease in the Americas: An ecohealth perspective. *Cad Saude Publ.* **2009**, *25* (Suppl. 1), S71–S82.
11. International Organization for Migration. Americas and the Caribbean: United Nations. 2020. Available online: https://www.iom.int/americas-and-caribbean (accessed on 15 April 2020).
12. Forsyth, C.J.; Hernandez, S.; Flores, C.A.; Roman, M.F.; Nieto, J.M.; Marquez, G.; Sequeira, J.; Sequeira, H.; Meymandi, S.K. "It's Like a Phantom Disease": Patient Perspectives on Access to Treatment for Chagas Disease in the United States. *Am. J. Trop. Med. Hyg.* **2018**, *98*, 735–741. [CrossRef] [PubMed]
13. Ventura-Garcia, L.; Roura, M.; Pell, C.; Posada, E.; Gascón, J.; Aldasoro, E.; Muñoz, J.; Pool, R. Socio-Cultural Aspects of Chagas Disease: A Systematic Review of Qualitative Research. *PLOS Negl. Trop. Dis.* **2013**, *7*, e2410. [CrossRef] [PubMed]
14. Jackson, Y.; Castillo, S.; Hammond, P.; Besson, M.; Brawand-Bron, A.; Urzola, D.; Gaspoz, J.M.; Chappuis, F. Metabolic, mental health, behavioural and socioeconomic characteristics of migrants with Chagas disease in a non-endemic country. *Trop. Med. Int. Health* **2012**, *17*, 595–603. [CrossRef] [PubMed]
15. United Nations. 2018 Revision of World Urbanization Prospects: Department of Economic and Social Affairs. 2018. Available online: https://www.un.org/development/desa/publications/2018-revision-of-world-urbanization-prospects.html (accessed on 15 April 2020).
16. Instituto Brasileiro de Geografia e Estatística. *Censo Demografico 2010: Resultados Gerais da Amostra*; IBGE: Rio de Janeiro, Brazil, 2012.
17. Balago, R. 'Hoje, os Bolivianos Investem em São Paulo', Afirma Cônsul-Geral da Bolívia. *Folha de S.Paulo.* 20 April 2013. Available online: https://m.folha.uol.com.br/saopaulo/2013/04/1265431-hoje-os-bolivianos-investem-em-sao-paulo-afirma-consul-geral-da-bolivia.shtml (accessed on 15 April 2020).
18. Souchaud, S.; Do Carmo, R.L.; Fusco, W. Mobilidade populacional e migração no Mercosul: A fronteira do Brasil com Bolívia e Paraguai. *Teor. Pesqui.* **2007**, *16*, 36–60.

19. Souchaud, S. A imigração boliviana em São Paulo. Deslocamentos e Reconstruções da Experiência Migrante, 2008, Rio de Janeiro, Brazil. Available online: https://halshs.archives-ouvertes.fr/file/index/docid/486059/filename/2010Souchaud_NIEM_ImigracaoBolivianaSaoPaulo_2009VersaoFinal.pdf (accessed on 15 April 2020).
20. Carballo, M.; Nerurkar, A. Migration, Refugees, and Health Risks. *Emerg. Infect. Dis.* **2001**, *7*, 556. [CrossRef] [PubMed]
21. Luna, E.J.; Furucho, C.R.; Silva, R.A.; Wanderley, D.M.; Carvalho, N.B.; Satolo, C.G.; Leite, R.M.; Silveira, C.; Silva, L.; Aith, F.M.; et al. Prevalence of *Trypanosoma cruzi* infection among Bolivian immigrants in the city of São Paulo, Brazil. *Mem. Inst. Osw. Cruz* **2017**, *112*, 70–74. [CrossRef]
22. Meymandi, S.K.; Forsyth, C.J.; Soverow, J.; Hernandez, S.; Sanchez, D.; Montgomery, S.P.; Traina, M. Prevalence of Chagas Disease in the Latin American-born Population of Los Angeles. *Clin. Infect. Dis.* **2017**, *64*, 1182–1188. [CrossRef]
23. Navarro, M.; Berens-Riha, N.; Hohnerlein, S.; Seiringer, P.; von Saldern, C.; Garcia, S.; Blasco-Hernández, T.; Navaza, B.; Shock, J.; Bretzel, G.; et al. Cross-sectional, descriptive study of Chagas disease among citizens of Bolivian origin living in Munich, Germany. *BMJ Open* **2017**, *7*, e013960. [CrossRef]
24. Pane, S.; Giancola, M.L.; Piselli, P.; Corpolongo, A.; Repetto, E.; Bellagamba, R.; Cimaglia, C.; Carrara, S.; Ghirga, P.; Oliva, A.; et al. Serological evaluation for Chagas disease in migrants from Latin American countries resident in Rome, Italy. *BMC Infect Dis.* **2018**, *18*, 212. [CrossRef]
25. Requena-Mendez, A.; Moore, D.A.; Subira, C.; Munoz, J. Addressing the neglect: Chagas disease in London, UK. *Lancet Glob. Health* **2016**, *4*, e231–e233. [CrossRef]
26. Rodolfo, A.K.-F.; Ivan, I.; Gabriela, R.; Francisco, C. Chagas disease prevalence in pregnant women: Migration and risk of congenital transmission. *J. Infect. Develop. Count.* **2016**, *10*, 895–901.
27. Muñoz, J.; i Prat, J.G.; Gállego, M.; Gimeno, F.; Treviño, B.; López-Chejade, P.; Ribera, O.; Molina, L.; Sanz, S.; Pinazo, M.J.; et al. Clinical profile of *Trypanosoma cruzi* infection in a non-endemic setting: Immigration and Chagas disease in Barcelona (Spain). *Acta Trop.* **2009**, *111*, 51–55. [CrossRef] [PubMed]
28. World Health Organization. *A Human Rights-Based Approach to Neglected Tropical Diseases*; WHO: Geneva, Switzerland, 2010; Available online: https://www.who.int/gender-equity-rights/knowledge/ntd-information-sheet-eng.pdf?ua=1 (accessed on 15 April 2020).
29. Yasuda, M.A.S.; Sátolo, C.G.; Carvalho, N.B.; Atala, M.M.; Ferrufino, R.Q.; Leite, R.M.; Furucho, C.R.; Luna, E.; Silva, R.A.; Hage, M.; et al. Interdisciplinary approach at the primary healthcare level for Bolivian immigrants with Chagas disease in the city of São Paulo. *PLOS Negl. Trop. Dis.* **2017**, *11*, e0005466.
30. Carneiro Junior, N.; Silveira, C.; Silva, L.M.B.; Shikanai-Yasuda, M.A. Migração boliviana e doença de Chagas: Limites na atuação do Sistema Único de Saúde brasileiro (SUS). *Interface Comun. Saúde Educ.* **2018**, *22*, 87–96. [CrossRef]
31. Presidencia da Republica, B. Lei 6.815 Define a situação jurídica do estrangeiro no Brasil, cria o Conselho Nacional de Imigração. Brasilia 1980. Available online: http://www.planalto.gov.br/ccivil_03/leis/l6815.htm (accessed on 22 February 2016).
32. Presidencia da Republica, B. Lei 11.961. Dispõe sobre a residência provisória para o estrangeiro em situação irregular no território nacional e dá outras providências. Brasilia. 2009. Available online: http://www.planalto.gov.br/ccivil_03/_Ato2007-2010/2009/Lei/L11961.htm (accessed on 15 April 2020).
33. Presidencia da Republica, B. Brasil Lei 12.401, de 28 de abril de 2011. Altera a Lei no 8.080, de 19 de setembro de 1990, para dispor sobre a assistência terapêutica e a incorporação de tecnologia em saúde no âmbito do Sistema Único de Saúde—SUS. Brasilia. 2011. Available online: http://www.planalto.gov.br/ccivil_03/_Ato2011-2014/2011/Lei/L12401.htm (accessed on 15 April 2020).
34. Ministério da Saúde. Portaria número 2.488 de 21 de outubro de 2011. Aprova a Polític a Nacional de Atenção Básica, estabelecendo a revisão de diretrizes e normas para a organização da Atenção Básica, para a Estratégia Saúde da Família (ESF) e o Programa de Agentes Comunitários de Saúde (PACS). Available online: https://bvsms.saude.gov.br/bvs/saudelegis/gm/2011/prt2488_21_10_2011.html (accessed on 15 April 2020).
35. Ministerio da Saude, B. Cadernos de Atenção Básica. Vigilância em Saúde: Zoonoses. Brasilia. 2009. Available online: http://189.28.128.100/dab/docs/publicacoes/cadernos_ab/abcad22.pdf (accessed on 15 April 2020).
36. Andrade, J.P.D.; Marin Neto, J.A.; De Paola, A.A.V.; Vilas-Boas, F.; Oliveira, G.M.M.; Bacal, F.; Bocchi, E.A.; Almeida, D.R.; Fragata Filho, A.A.; Moreira, M.D.C.V.; et al. I Latin American Guidelines for the diagnosis and treatment of Chagas' heart disease: Executive summary. *Arq. Bras Cardiol.* **2011**, *96*, 434–442. [CrossRef]

37. Pan American Health Organization. Guia Para Vigilância, Prevenção, Controle e Manejo Clínico da Doença de Chagas Aguda Transmitida por Alimentos. 2009. Available online: http://bvsms.saude.gov.br/bvs/publicacoes/guia_vigilancia_prevencao_doenca_chagas.pdf (accessed on 15 April 2020).
38. Ministério da Saúde, B. Protocolo de Doença de Chagas. In: Secretaria de Ciência Tecnologia e Insumos Estratégicos, Portaria número 57, editor. Brasilia. 2018. Available online: http://conitec.gov.br/images/PCDT_Doenca_de_Chagas.pdf (accessed on 15 April 2020).
39. Morillo, C.A.; Marin-Neto, J.A.; Avezum, A.; Sosa-Estani, S.; Rassi, A., Jr.; Rosas, F.; Villena, E.; Quiroz, R.; Bonilla, R.; Britto, C.; et al. Randomized Trial of Benznidazole for Chronic Chagas' Cardiomyopathy. *N. Engl. J. Med.* **2015**, *373*, 1295–1306. [CrossRef]
40. Cardoso, C.S.; Ribeiro, A.L.P.; Oliveira, C.D.L.; Oliveira, L.C.; Ferreira, A.M.; Bierrenbach, A.L.; Silva, J.L.P.; Colosimo, E.A.; Ferreira, J.E.; Lee, T.H.; et al. Beneficial effects of benznidazole in Chagas disease: NIH SaMi-Trop cohort study. *PLOS Negl. Trop. Dis.* **2018**, *12*, e0006814. [CrossRef]
41. Fabbro, D.L.; Streiger, M.L.; Arias, E.D.; Bizai, M.L.; del Barco, M.; Amicone, N.A. Trypanocide treatment among adults with chronic Chagas disease living in Santa Fe city (Argentina), over a mean follow-up of 21 years: Parasitological, serological and clinical evolution. *Rev. Soc. Bras Med. Trop.* **2007**, *40*, 1–10. [CrossRef]
42. Viotti, R.; Vigliano, C.; Lococo, B.; Bertocchi, G.; Petti, M.; Alvarez, M.G.; Postan, M.; Armenti, A. Long-term cardiac outcomes of treating chronic Chagas disease with benznidazole versus no treatment: A nonrandomized trial. *Ann. Int. Med.* **2006**, *144*, 724–734. [CrossRef]
43. Sosa Estani, S.; Segura, E.L.; Ruiz, A.M.; Velazquez, E.; Porcel, B.M.; Yampotis, C. Efficacy of chemotherapy with benznidazole in children in the indeterminate phase of Chagas' disease. *Am. J. Trop. Med. Hyg.* **1998**, *59*, 526–529. [CrossRef]
44. Alonso-Vega, C.; Billot, C.; Torrico, F. Achievements and challenges upon the implementation of a program for national control of congenital Chagas in Bolivia: Results 2004–2009. *PLoS Negl. Trop. Dis.* **2013**, *7*, e2304. [CrossRef] [PubMed]
45. Martins-Melo, F.R.; Lima, M.D.S.; Ramos, A.N., Jr.; Alencar, C.H.; Heukelbach, J. Systematic review: Prevalence of Chagas disease in pregnant women and congenital transmission of *Trypanosoma cruzi* in Brazil: A systematic review and meta-analysis. *Trop. Med. Int. Health* **2014**, *19*, 943–957. [CrossRef] [PubMed]
46. Repetto, E.C.; Zachariah, R.; Kumar, A.; Angheben, A.; Gobbi, F.; Anselmi, M.; Al Rousan, A.; Torrico, C.; Ruiz, R.; Ledezma, G.; et al. Neglect of a Neglected Disease in Italy: The Challenge of Access-to-Care for Chagas Disease in Bergamo Area. *PLOS Negl. Trop. Dis.* **2015**, *9*, e0004103. [CrossRef] [PubMed]
47. Jackson, Y.; Varcher Herrera, M.; Gascon, J. Economic crisis and increased immigrant mobility: New challenges in managing Chagas disease in Europe. *Bull World Health Organ.* **2014**, *92*, 771–772. [CrossRef]
48. Waldman, M.T.C. Movimentos migratórios; sob a perspectiva do direito à saúde; imigrantes bolivianos em São Paulo. *Rev. Direito Sanit. São Paulo* **2011**, *2*, 90–114. [CrossRef]

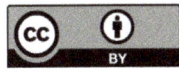

© 2020 by the authors. Licensee MDPI, Basel, Switzerland. This article is an open access article distributed under the terms and conditions of the Creative Commons Attribution (CC BY) license (http://creativecommons.org/licenses/by/4.0/).

pieces of evidence of sexual recombination in *T. cruzi* populations from Brazil, Peru, Ecuador, and Colombia.

A different aspect of sexual or parasexual exchanges in *T. cruzi* has to do with the inheritance of mitochondrial DNA. The kinetoplast, a DNA body common to all Kinetoplastida, is an intricate mesh of mini and maxicircles; the former participate in the editing process of the encrypted genes encoded in the maxicircle, which is the equivalent of the mitochondrial DNA in other organisms. There are claims of the uniparental contribution of K-DNA in parasexual hybrids [23,66] but with pieces of evidence of exchanges with other clades or DTUs. Little is known about how these inter-DTUs introgression processes occur [30,67,68].

Many questions about sexuality remain, such as when and where sexual recombination occurs? Are gametes ever produced? Are both gametes contributing with mitochondrial DNA, in which differentiation forms, and in which host does it take place?

5. Clonal or Not Clonal, is That the Question?

A panmictic evolution with sexual exchanges through gametes or parasexual fusion of cells [5,69] does not appear to contradict the general hypothesis that the *T. cruzi* population structure appears to be clonal [69,70], or as more recently coined, has a predominantly clonal signal [70]. Either way, the apparent infrequency of sexual exchanges indicates it is not obligatory for *T. cruzi*. Clonality can result from genome instability since aneuplody and variable gene copy numbers could be obstacles for efficient meiotic recombination. However, under challenging situations, this instability can generate gene variants with adaptive advantages at a faster rate when compared to sexual recombination. This fact agrees with the low frequency of sexual recombination registered in whole genomic analysis or the limited recombination between hybrid strain chromosomes [23,34,70]. Sexual recombination has been detected mainly in closely related populations, and rarely between strains from different near-clades. Some authors claim that sexual recombination occurs more frequently but remains undetected because it happens in closely related parasites (endogamy) [40]. The key to alternatives ways of evolution may reside in the heterogeneity of *T. cruzi* populations, which even under in vitro culturing are very heterogeneous [71,72]. Within the population, some members may retain the ability for sexual exchanges, while the majority stays clonal and adapted to a given environment. The accumulation of deleterious mutations during clonal propagation may drive a cell to its death and be eliminated from the population (Muller Rachet) [73]. However, since *T. cruzi* populations do not divide synchronously, not all cells will reach this end simultaneously, and some of the survivors with fewer genome alterations or those that have reversed to the diploid [30] condition by chromosomal loss, can engage in sexual or parasexual exchanges to replenish population fitness. Although it has been suggested that sexual recombination occurs inside the vertebrate host [68], it seems to the parasite's advantage to be able to generate variants at all stages of differentiation, as well as in all hosts, so populations can go either way, panmictic or clonal.

Genome-wise, *T. cruzi* seems to be the master of variation, a property that explains its resilience, its capacity to infect a wide range of hosts and vectors, the utilization of multiple ways of infection, its capacity to recover its karyotype after a massive Gamma ray irradiations [74], and the rapid acquisition of surface protein variants to escape the host's immune system, a fact that makes the attainment of an effective vaccine very difficult.

6. Final Considerations

One indisputable fact is that despite the many genetic variations and polymorphisms recorded among *T. cruzi* strains, the parasite is a pathogenic entity that keeps its basic cell architecture and differentiation programs and infects humans causing Chagas disease. For practitioners, infections by *T. cruzi*, regardless of the considerations about the parasite types, are treated in the same classical way, which involves the drugs nifurtimox or benznidazol.

Nonetheless, the information provided by the 2005 publication paved the way for the generation of new diagnostic tools, the discovery of important metabolic routes, the publication of nearly 2000 research papers, and the production of a wealth of information that allows a more systemic approach to *T. cruzi* biology and a large scale search for druggable targets [75–77].

The genetic experimentation with *T. cruzi* has lagged behind *Leishmania* and *T. brucei* due to the lack of cloning vectors with inducible promoters and/or an RNAi machinery that could allow for checking the importance and function of genes, and although the recent use of CRISPR technologies has facilitated this task [78,79], we are far from what is known about *T. brucei*. A more in-depth insight into the causes of *T. cruzi* genome plasticity and genetic variability may lead to understanding how the parasite generates diversity and provide us with better tools to effectively tackle Chagas disease.

Last, but certainly not least, the Trypanosomatid genomes contributed to the generation of a new cohort of young LA researchers in genomics and bioinformatics, some of whom are currently successfully engaged in fighting other diseases.

Funding: This research receives no external funding.

Conflicts of Interest: The authors declare no conflict of interest.

References

1. WHO. *Chagas Disease (American Trypanosomiasis)*; WHO: Geneva, Switzerland, 2019. Available online: https://www.who.int/health-topics/chagas-disease#tab=tab_1 (accessed on 27 June 2020).
2. Lidani, K.C.F.; Andrade, F.A.; Bavia, L.; Damasceno, F.S.; Beltrame, M.H.; Messias-Reason, I.J.; Sandri, T.L. Chagas Disease: From Discovery to a Worldwide Health Problem. *Front. Public Health* **2019**, *7*, 166. [CrossRef] [PubMed]
3. De Noya, B.A.; Colmenares, C.; Díaz-Bello, Z.; Ruiz-Guevara, R.; Medina, K.; Muñoz-Calderón, A.; Mauriello, L.; Cabrerad, E.; Montiel, L.; Losada, S.; et al. Orally-transmitted Chagas disease: Epidemiological, clinical, serological and molecular outcomes of a school microepidemic in Chichiriviche de la Costa, Venezuela. *Parasite Epidemiol. Control* **2016**, 2405–6731. [CrossRef]
4. Zingales, B. *Trypanosoma cruzi* genetic diversity: Something new for something known about Chagas disease manifestations, serodiagnosis, and drug sensitivity. *Acta Trop.* **2018**, *184*, 38–52. [CrossRef]
5. Ramirez, J.D.; Llewellyn, M.S. Reproductive clonality in protozoan pathogens—Truth or artefact? *Mol. Ecol.* **2014**, *23*, 4195–4202. [CrossRef]
6. International Human Genome Consortium Initial. Sequencing and Analysis of the Human Genome. *Nature* **2001**, *409*, 860–921. [CrossRef] [PubMed]
7. Angier, N. Great 15'year Project to decipher Genes stirs opposition. *The New York Times. Science Times*, 15 June 1990.
8. The human Genome. *Deciphering the Blueprint of Heredity*; Cooper, N.G., Ed.; University Science Books: Mill Valley, CA, USA, 1994; ISBN 0-935702-29-6.
9. Latham, L. The failure of the genome. *The Guardian*, 17 April 2011.
10. Ramsey, J.M.; Schofield, C.J. Control of Chagas disease vectors. *Salud Publica Mex.* **2003**, *45*, 123–128. [CrossRef]
11. Venter, J.C.; Adams, M.D.; Myers, E.W.; Li, P.W.; Mural, R.J.; Smith, H.O.; Yandell, M.; Evans, C.A.; Holt, R.A.; Gocayne, J.D.; et al. The sequence of human genome. *Science* **2001**, *291*, 1304–1351. [CrossRef]
12. Degrave, W.; Levin, M.J.; Franco da Silveira, J.; Morel, C.M. Parasite Genome Projects and the *Trypanosoma cruzi* Genome Initiative. *Mem. Inst. Oswaldo Cruz* **1997**, *92*, 859–862. [CrossRef]
13. Simpson, A.J.; Reinach, F.C.; Arruda, P.; Abreu, F.A.; Acencio, M.; Alvarenga, R.; Alves, L.M.; Araya, J.E.; Baia, G.S.; Baptista, C.S.; et al. The *Xylella fastidiosa* Consortium of the Organization for Nucleotide Sequencing and Analysis The genome sequence of the plant pathogen *Xylella fastidiosa*. *Nature* **2000**, *406*, 151–157. [CrossRef]
14. Ferrari, I.; Lorenzi, H.; Santos, M.R.; Brandariz, S.; Requena, J.M.; Schijman, A.; Vázquez, M.; Silveira, J.F.; Ben-Dov, C.; Medrano, S.; et al. Towards the Physical Map of the *Trypanosoma cruzi* Nuclear Genome: Construction of YAC and BAC Libraries of the Reference Clone *T. cruzi* CL-Brener. *Mem. Inst. Oswaldo Cruz* **1997**, *92*, 843–852. [CrossRef]

15. Morel, C.M.; Acharya, T.; Broun, D.; Dangi, A.; Elias, C.; Ganguly, N.K.; Gardner, C.A.; Gupta, R.K.; Haycock, J.; Heher, A.D.; et al. Health Innovation Networks to Help Developing Countries Address Neglected Diseases. *Science* **2005**, *309*, 401–404. [CrossRef]
16. The *Trypanosoma cruzi* Genome Consortium. The *Trypanosoma cruzi* Genome Initiative. *Parasitol. Today* **1997**, *1*, 16–21. [CrossRef]
17. Cano, M.I.; Gruber, A.; Vazquez, M.; Cortés, A.; Levin, M.J.; González, A.; Degrave, W.; Rondinelli, E.; Zingales, B.; Ramirez, J.L.; et al. Molecular karyotype of clone CL Brener chosen for the *Trypanosoma cruzi* Genome Project. *Mol. Biochem. Parasitol.* **1995**, *71*, 273–278. [CrossRef]
18. Henriksson, J.; Aslund, L.; Petersson, U. Karyotype variability in *Trypanosoma cruzi*. *Parasitol. Today* **1996**, *12*, 108–114. [CrossRef]
19. Santos, M.R.; Lorenzi, H.; Porcile, P.; Carmo, M.S.; Schijman, A.; Brandão, A.; Araya, J.E.; Gomes, H.B.; Chiurillo, M.A.; Ramirez, J.L.; et al. Physical mapping of a 670-kb region of chromosomes XVI and XVII from the human protozoan parasite *Trypanosoma cruzi* encompassing the genes for two Immunodominant antigens. *Genome Res.* **1999**, *9*, 1268–1276. [CrossRef] [PubMed]
20. Bringaud, F.; Biteau, N.; Melville, S.E.; Hez, S.; El-Sayed, N.M. A New, Expressed Multigene Family Containing a Hot Spot for Insertion of Retroelements are associated with Polymorphic Subtelomeric Regions of *Trypanosoma brucei*. *Eukaryot Cell* **2002**, *1*, 137–151. [CrossRef] [PubMed]
21. Olivares, M.; Thomas, M.C.; Lopez-Barajas, A.; Requena, J.M.; Garcia-Perez, J.L.; Angel, S. Genome clustering of the *Trypanosoma cruzi* nonlong Terminal L1Tc retrotransposon with defined intersperse repeated DNA elements. *Electrophoresis* **2000**, *21*, 2973–2982. [CrossRef]
22. Chiurillo, M.A.; Santos, M.R.M.; Da Silveira, J.F.; Ramírez, J.L. An improved general approach for cloning and characterizing telomeres: The protozoan parasite *Trypanosoma cruzi* as model organism. *Gene* **1999**, *294*, 197–204. [CrossRef]
23. El-Sayed, N.M.; Myler, P.J.; Bartholomeu, D.C.; Nilsson, D.; Aggarwal, G.; Tran, N.H.; Ghedin, E.; Worthey, E.A.; Delcher, A.L.; Blandin, G.; et al. The Genome Sequence of *Trypanosoma cruzi*, Etiologic Agent of Chagas Disease. *Science* **2005**, *309*, 409–415. [CrossRef]
24. El-Sayed, N.M.; Myler, P.J.; Blandin, G.; Berriman, M.; Crabtree, J.; Aggarwal, G.; Caler, E.; Renauld, H.; Worthey, E.A.; Hertz-Fowleret, C.; et al. Comparative genomics of trypanosomatid parasitic protozoa. *Science* **2005**, *309*, 404–409. [CrossRef]
25. Olivares, M.; López, M.C.; García-Pérez, J.L.; Briones, P.; Pulgar, M.; Thomas, M.C. The endonuclease NL1Tc encoded by the LINE L1Tc from *Trypanosoma cruzi* protects parasites from daunorubicin DNA damage. *Biochim. Biophys. Acta* **2003**, *1626*, 25–32. [CrossRef]
26. Kim, D.; Chiurillo, M.A.; El-Sayed, N.; Jones, K.; Santos, M.R.; Porcile, P.E.; Andersson, B.; Myler, P.; da Silveira, J.F.; Ramírez, J.L. Telomere and subtelomere of *Trypanosoma cruzi* chromosomes are enriched in (pseudo)genes of retrotransposon hot spot and trans-sialidase-like gene families: The origins of *T. cruzi* telomeres. *Gene* **2005**, *346*, 53–161. [CrossRef]
27. Atwood, J.A., III; Weatherly, D.B.; Minning, T.A.; Bundy, B.; Cavola, C.; Opperdoes, F.R.; Orlando, R.; Tarleton, R.L. The *Trypanosoma cruzi* Proteome. *Science* **2005**, *309*, 473–476. [CrossRef] [PubMed]
28. Roberts, S.B.; Robichaux, J.L.; Chavali, K.; Manque, P.A.; Lee, V.; Lara, A.M.; Manque, P.A.; Lee, V.; Lara, M.A.; Papin, J.A.; et al. Proteomic and network analysis characterize stage-specific metabolism in *Trypanosoma cruzi*. *BMC Syst. Biol.* **2009**, *3*, 52. [CrossRef] [PubMed]
29. Carrea, A.; Diambra, L. Systems Biology Approach to Model the Life Cycle of *Trypanosoma cruzi*. *PLoS ONE* **2016**, *11*, e0146947. [CrossRef] [PubMed]
30. Reis-Cunha, J.L.; Baptista, R.P.; Rodriguez-Luiz, G.F.; Coquiero-dos-santos, A.; Valdivia, H.O.; Cardoso, M.S.; D'Ávila, D.A.; Dias, F.; Fujiwara, R.T.; Galvão, L.; et al. Whole genome sequencing of *Trypanosoma cruzi* field Isolates reveal extensive genomic variability and complex aneuploidy patterns within TcII DTU. *BMC Genom.* **2018**, *19*, 816. [CrossRef]
31. Falconer, E.; Hills, M.; Naumann, U.; Poon, S.; Chavez, E.A.; Sanders, A.D.; Zhao, Y.; Hirst, M.; Lansdorp, P.M. DNA template strand sequencing of single cells maps genomic rearrangements at high resolution. *Nat. Methods* **2012**, *9*, 1107–1112. [CrossRef]
32. Sanders, A.D.; Falconer, E.; Hills, M.; Spierings, D.C.J.; Lansdor, P.M. Single-cell template strand sequencing by Strand-seq the characterization of individual homologs. *Nat. Prot.* **2017**, *712*, 1151–1176. [CrossRef]

33. Weatherly, D.B.; Boehlke, C.; Tarleton, R.L. Chromosome level assembly of the hybrid *Trypanosoma cruzi* genome. *BMC Genom.* **2009**, *10*, 255. [CrossRef]
34. Frazen, O.; Ochaya, S.; Sherwood, E.; Lewis, M.D.; Llewellyn, M.S.; Miles, M.A.; Anderson, B. Shotgun Sequencing Analysis of *Trypanosoma cruzi* I Sylvio X10/1 and comparison with *T. cruzi* VI CL Brener. *PLoS Negl. Trop. Dis.* **2011**, *5*, e984. [CrossRef]
35. Callejas-Hernandez, F.; Rastrojo, A.; Poveda, C.; Girones, N.; Fresno, M. Genomic assemblies of newly sequenced *Trypanosoma cruzi* strains reveal new genomic expansion and greater complexity. *Sci. Rep.* **2018**, *8*, 14631. [CrossRef] [PubMed]
36. Berna, L.; Rodriguez, M.; Chiribao, M.L.; Parodi-Talice, A.; Pita, S.; Rijo, G.; Alvarez-Valin, F.; Robello, C. Expanding an expanded Genome long-read sequencing of *Trypanosoma cruzi* genome. *Microb. Genom.* **2018**, *4*. [CrossRef] [PubMed]
37. Talavera-Lopez, C.; Messenger, L.A.; Lewis, M.D.; Yeo, M.; Reis-Cunha, J.L.; Bartholomeu, D.C.; Calzada, J.E.; Saldaña, A.; Ramírez, J.D.; Guhl, F. Repeat-driven generation of antigenic diversity in a major human pathogen, *Trypanosoma cruzi*. *bioRxiv* **2018**. [CrossRef]
38. Bradwell, K.R.; Koparde, V.N.; Matveyev, A.V.; Serrano, M.G.; Alves, J.; Parikh, H.; Huang, B.; Lee, V.; Espinosa-Alvarez, O.; Ortiz, P.A.; et al. Genomic comparison of Trypanosoma conorhini and Trypanosoma rangeli to Trypanosoma cruzi strains of high and low virulence. *BMC Genom.* **2018**, *19*, 770. [CrossRef] [PubMed]
39. Berry, A.S.F.; Salazar-Sánchez, R.; Castillo-Neyra, R.; Borrini-Mayorí, K.; Chipana-Ramos, C.; Vargas-Maquera, M.; Ancca-Juarez, J.; Náquira-Velarde, C.; Levy, M.Z.; Brisson, D. Sexual reproduction in a natural *Trypanosoma cruzi* population. *PLoS Negl. Trop. Dis.* **2019**, *13*, e0007392. [CrossRef]
40. Lewis, M.; Llewellyn, M.S.; Yeo, M.; Acosta, N.; Gaunt, M.W.; Miles, M.A. Recent, Independent and Anthropogenic Origins of *Trypanosoma cruzi* Hybrids. *PLos Negl. Trop. Dis.* **2011**, *5*, e1363. [CrossRef]
41. Messenger, L.A.; Miles, M.A. Evidence and importance of genetic exchange among field populations of *Trypanosoma cruzi*. *Acta Trop.* **2015**, *151*, 150–155. [CrossRef]
42. Schwabl, P.; Imamura, H.; Van den Broeck, F.; Costales, J.A.; Maiguashca-Sánchez, J.; Miles, M.A.; Andersson, B.; Grijalva, M.J.; Llewellyn, M.S. Meiotic sex in Chagas disease parasite *Trypanosoma cruzi*. *Nat. Commun.* **2019**, *10*, 3972. [CrossRef]
43. Minning, D.; Weatherly, B.; Flibotte, S.; Tarleton, R.L. Widespread, focal copy Number variations (CNV)and whole chromosome aneuploidies in *Trypanosoma cruzi* Strains revealed by array comparative genomic hybridization. *BMC Genom.* **2011**, *12*, 139. [CrossRef]
44. De Pablos, L.M.; Osuna, A. Multigene Families in *Trypanosoma cruzi* and Their Role in Infectivity. *Infect. Immun.* **2012**, *7*, 2258–2264. [CrossRef]
45. Cardoso, M.S.; Reis-Cunha, J.L.; Bartholomeu, D.C. Evasion of the Immune Response by *Trypanosoma cruzi* during Acute Infection. *Front. Immunol.* **2016**, *6*, 659. [CrossRef]
46. Sheltzer, J.M.; Blank, H.M.; Pfau, S.J.; Tange, Y.; George, B.M.; Humpton, T.J.; Brito, I.L.; Hiraoka, Y.; Niwa, O.; Amon, A. Aneuploidy drives genomic instability in yeast. *Science* **2011**, *333*, 1026–1030. [CrossRef] [PubMed]
47. Polakova, S.; Blume, C.; Zárate, J.A.; Mentel, M.; Jørck-Ramberg, D.; Stenderup, J.; Piskur, J. Formation of new chromosomes as a virulence mechanism in yeast *Candida glabrata*. *PNAS* **2009**, *106*, 2688–2693. [CrossRef] [PubMed]
48. Reis-Cunha, J.L.; Rodrigues-Luiz, G.F.; Valdivia, H.O.; Baptista, R.P.; Mendes, T.A.; de Morais, G.L.; Macedo, A.M.; Bern, C.; Gilman, R.H. Chromosomal copy Number variation reveals differential levels of genomic plasticity in distinct *Trypanosoma cruzi* strains. *BMC Genom.* **2015**, *16*, 499. [CrossRef]
49. Briones, M.R.; Egima, C.M.; Eichinger, D.; Schenkman, S. Trans-sialidase genes expressed in mammalian forms of *Trypanosoma cruzi* evolved from ancestor genes expressed in insect forms of the parasite. *J. Mol. Evol.* **1995**, *41*, 120–131. [CrossRef] [PubMed]
50. Chiurillo, M.A.; Cortez, D.R.; Lima, F.M.; Cortez, C.; Ramírez, J.L.; Martins, A.G.; Serrano, M.G.; Teixeira, M.M.; da Silveira, J.F. The diversity and expansion of the trans-sialidase gene family is a common feature in *Trypanosoma cruzi* clade members. *Infect. Genet. Evol.* **2016**, *37*, 266–274. [CrossRef] [PubMed]
51. Frasch, A.C. Functional diversity in the trans-sialidase and mucin families in *Trypanosoma cruzi*. *Parasitol. Today* **2000**, *16*, 282–286. [CrossRef]
52. Yoshida, N. *Trypanosoma cruzi* infection by oral route, how the interplay between parasite and host components modulate infectivity. *Parasitol. Int.* **2008**, *57*, 105–109. [CrossRef]

53. Freitas, L.M.; dos Santos, S.L.; Rodrigues-Luiz, G.F.; Mendes, T.A.; Rodrigues, T.S.; Gazzinelli, R.T.; Teixeira, S.M.; Fujiwara, R.T.; Bartholomeu, D.C. Genomic analyses, gene expression and antigenic profile of the trans-sialidase superfamily of *Trypanosoma cruzi* reveal an undetected level of complexity. *PLoS ONE* **2011**, *6*, e25914. [CrossRef] [PubMed]
54. Maeda, F.Y.; Clemente, T.M.; Macedo, S.; Cortez, C.; Yoshida, N. Host cell invasion and oral infection by *Trypanosoma cruzi* strains of genetic groups TcI and TcIV from chagasic patients. *Parasites Vectors* **2016**, *9*, 189. [CrossRef]
55. Azuaje, F.; Ramirez, J.L.; Da Silveira, J.F. In silico, biologically inspired modelling of genomic variation generation in surface proteins of *Trypanosoma cruzi*. *Kinetoplastid Biol. Dis.* **2007**, *6*, 6. [CrossRef]
56. Reynaud, C.A.; Anquez, V.; Grimal, H.; Weill, J.C. A hyperconversion mechanism generates the chicken light chain preimmune repertoire. *Cell* **1987**, *48*, 379–388. [CrossRef]
57. Thon, G.; Baltz, T.; Eisen, H. Antigenic diversity by the recombination of pseudogenes. *Genes Dev.* **1989**, *3*, 1247–1254. [CrossRef] [PubMed]
58. Allen, C.L.; Kelly, J.M. *Trypanosoma cruzi*: Mucin pseudogenes organized in a tandem array. *Exp. Parasitol.* **2001**, *97*, 173–177. [CrossRef] [PubMed]
59. Wen, Y.Z.; Zheng, L.L.; Qu, L.H.; Ayala, F.J.; Lun, Z.R. Pseudogenes are not pseudo any more. *RNA Biol.* **2012**, *9*, 27–32. [CrossRef] [PubMed]
60. Macías, F.; Afonso-Lehmann, R.; López, M.C.; Gómez, I.; Thomas, M.C. Biology of *Trypanosoma cruzi* Retrotransposons: From an Enzymatic to a Structural Point of View. *Curr. Genom.* **2018**, *19*, 110–118. [CrossRef] [PubMed]
61. Chiurillo, M.A.; Moraes Barros, R.R.; Souza, R.T.; Marini, M.M.; Antonio, C.R.; Cortez, D.R.; Curto, M.Á.; Lorenzi, H.A.; Schijman, A.G.; Ramirez, J.L.; et al. Subtelomeric I-SceI-Mediated Double-Strand Breaks Are Repaired by Homologous Recombination in *Trypanosoma cruzi*. *Front. Microbiol.* **2016**, *7*, 2041. [CrossRef] [PubMed]
62. Moraes Barros, R.R.; Marini, M.M.; Antônio, C.R.; Cortez, D.R.; Miyake, A.M.; Lima, F.M.; Ruiz, J.C.; Bartholomeu, D.C.; Chiurillo, M.A.; Ramirez, J.L.; et al. Anatomy and evolution of telomeric and subtelomeric regions in the human protozoan parasite *Trypanosoma cruzi*. *BMC Genom.* **2012**, *13*, 229. [CrossRef]
63. Chiurillo, M.A.; Antonio, C.R.; Mendes Marini, M.; Torres de Souza, R.; Da Silveira, J.F. Chromosomes ends and the telomere biology in Trypanosomatids. *Front. Parasitol.* **2017**, *1*, 104–133. [CrossRef]
64. Ramirez, J.L. An Evolutionary View of *Trypanosoma cruzi* Telomeres. *Front. Cell. Infect. Microbiol.* **2020**, *9*, 439. [CrossRef]
65. Xing, J.; Wan, G.; Belancio, V.P.; Cordaux, R.; Deininger, P.L.; Batzer, M.A. Emergence of primate genes by retrotransposon mediated sequence transduction. *PNAS* **2006**, *103*, 17608–17613. [CrossRef] [PubMed]
66. Messenger, L.A.; Llewellyn, M.S.; Bhattacharyya, T.; Franzén, O.; Lewis, M.D.; Ramírez, J.D.; Carrasco, H.J.; Andersson, B.; Miles, M.A. Multiple mitochondrial Introgression events and heteroplasmy in *Trypanosoma cruzi* revealed by maxicircle MLST and next generation sequencing. *PLoS Negl. Trop. Dis.* **2012**, *6*, e1584. [CrossRef] [PubMed]
67. Rusman, F.; Floridia-Yapur, N.; Ragone, P.G.; Diosque, P.; Tomasini, N. Evidence of hybridization, mitochondrial introgression and biparental inheritance of the kDNA minicircles in *Trypanosoma cruzi* I. *PLoS Negl. Trop. Dis.* **2020**, *14*, e0007770. [CrossRef] [PubMed]
68. Gaunt, M.; Yeo, M.; Frame, I.; Stothard, J.R.; Carrasco, H.J.; Taylor, M.C.; Mena, S.S.; Veazey, P.; Miles, G.A.; Acosta, N. Mechanism of genetic exchange in American trypanosomes. *Nature* **2003**, *421*, 936–939. [CrossRef] [PubMed]
69. Tybairenc, M.; Kjellberg, F.; Ayala, F.J. A clonal theory of parasitic protozoa: The population structures of *Entamoeba*, *Giardia*, *Leishmania*, *Naegleria*, *Plasmodium*, *Trichomonas*, and *Trypanosoma* and their medical and taxonomical consequences. *PNAS* **1990**, *87*, 2414–2418. [CrossRef]
70. Tibayrenc, M.; Ayala, F.J. Genomics and High-Resolution Typing Confirm Predominant Clonal Evolution Down to a Microevolutionary Scale in *Trypanosoma cruzi*. *Pathogens* **2020**, *9*, 356. [CrossRef]
71. Seco-Hidalgo, V.; De Pablos, L.M.; Osuna, A. Transcriptional and phenotypical heterogeneity of *Trypanosoma cruzi* cell populations. *Open Biol.* **2015**, *5*, 150190. [CrossRef]
72. Muñoz-Calderón, A.; Díaz-Bello, Z.; Ramírez, J.L.; Noya, O.; de Noya, B.A. Nifurtimox response of *Trypanosoma cruzi* isolates from an outbreak of Chagas disease in Caracas, Venezuela. *J. Vector Borne Dis.* **2019**, *57*. [CrossRef]

73. Muller, H.J. Some aspects of sex. *Am. Nat.* **1932**, *703*, 118–138. [CrossRef]
74. Garcia, J.B.; Rocha, J.P.; Costa-Silva, H.M.; Alves, C.L.; Machado, C.R.; Cruz, A.K. *Leishmania major* and *Trypanosoma cruzi* present distinct DNA damage responses. *Mol. Biochem. Parasitol.* **2016**, *207*, 23–32. [CrossRef]
75. Donelson, J. The promise of *T. cruzi* genomics. *Nature* **2010**, *465*, S16–S17.
76. Bartholomeu, D.C.; Buck, G.A.; Teixeira, S.M.R.; El-Sayed, N.M.A. Genetics of Trypanosoma cruzi Nuclear Genome. In *American Trypanosomiasis Chagas Disease Chagas Disease One Hundred Years of Research*; Telleria, J., Tybayrenc, M., Eds.; Elsevier: Amsterdam, The Netherlands, 2010; pp. 433–448. ISBN 9780128010693.
77. Menezes, C.; Carneiro Costa, G.; Gollob, K.J.; Dutra, W.O. Clinical aspects of Chagas disease and implications for novel therapies. *Drug Dev. Res.* **2011**, *72*, 471–479. [CrossRef] [PubMed]
78. Soares Medeiros, L.C.; South, L.; Peng, D.; Bustamante, J.M.; Wang, W.; Bunkofske, M.; Perumal, N.; Sanchez-Valdez, F.; Tarleton, R.L. Rapid, Selection-Free, High-Efficiency Genome Editing in Protozoan Parasites Using CRISPR-Cas9 Ribonucleoproteins. *mBio* **2017**, *8*, e01788-17. [CrossRef]
79. Lander, N.; Li, Z.H.; Niyogi, S.; Docampo, R. CRISPR/Cas9-Induced Disruption of Paraflagellar Rod Protein 1 and 2 Genes in *Trypanosoma cruzi* Reveals Their Role in Flagellar Attachment. *mBio* **2015**, *6*, e01012-15. [CrossRef] [PubMed]

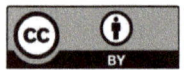

© 2020 by the author. Licensee MDPI, Basel, Switzerland. This article is an open access article distributed under the terms and conditions of the Creative Commons Attribution (CC BY) license (http://creativecommons.org/licenses/by/4.0/).

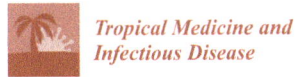

Review

Chagas Disease Infection Reactivation after Heart Transplant

Maria da Consolação Vieira Moreira [1] and José Renan Cunha-Melo [2,*]

1. School of Medicine, Federal University of Minas Gerais (UFMG), Av. Alfredo Balena 190, Belo Horizonte CEP 30130-110, MG, Brazil; mariacvmoreira@gmail.com
2. Department of Surgery, School of Medicine, Federal University of Minas Gerais (UFMG), Av. Alfredo Balena 190, Belo Horizonte CEP 30130-110, MG, Brazil
* Correspondence: jrcmelo@medicina.ufmg.br

Received: 8 May 2020; Accepted: 10 June 2020; Published: 29 June 2020

Abstract: Chagas disease, caused by a *Trypanosona cruzi* infection, is one of the main causes of heart failure in Latin America. It was originally a health problem endemic to South America, predominantly affecting residents of poor rural areas. With globalization and increasing migratory flows from these areas to large cities, the immigration of *T. cruzi* chronically-infected people to developed, non-endemic countries has occurred. This issue has emerged as an important consideration for heart transplant professionals. Currently, Chagas patients with end-stage heart failure may need a heart transplantation (HTx). This implies that in post-transplant immunosuppression therapy to avoid rejection in the recipient, there is the possibility of *T. cruzi* infection reactivation, increasing the morbidity and mortality rates. The management of heart transplant recipients due to Chagas disease requires awareness for early recognition and parasitic treatment of *T. cruzi* infection reactivation. This issue poses challenges for heart transplant professionals, especially regarding the differential diagnosis between rejection and reactivation episodes. The aim of this review is to discuss the complexity of the Chagas disease reactivation phenomenon in patients submitted to HTx for end-stage chagasic cardiomyopathy.

Keywords: chagasic cardiomyopathy; heart transplantation; Chagas disease reactivation; cardiac allograft rejection; treatment of reactivation

1. Brief Historical Context

The first human heart transplantation (HTx) was performed by Christian Barnard in December 1967 [1]. The patient was treated for rejection and died 18 days after HTx due to pneumonia and sepsis [2]. The available data today show that, in spite of fantastic scientific and technological developments, the problems of rejection, infection, allograft failure, cardiac allograft vasculopathy (CAV), and Chagas reactivation still constitute major problems faced by heart transplant centers.

The introduction of new immunosuppressive agents, such as cyclosporine A in 1980 and FK 506 (tacrolimus) in 1989, improved survival rates for all heart transplant recipients and definitively qualified HTx as the treatment of choice for end-stage heart failure [3]. In addition, advances in donor procurement, surgical techniques, post-HTx care, organ preservation, and the big jump in technological development (bringing great positive impacts in anesthesia, surgical interventions, and immunosuppression protocols), in conjunction with the accumulated experience at heart transplant institutions, have contributed to a great decrease in acute rejection episodes and an improvement of the overall results of HTx [3]. However, the donor shortage is still a worldwide problem [4]. To overcome this difficulty, the concept of donation after circulatory death donors and the extended criteria donors have been used as mechanisms to increase the donor pool [5,6]. Currently, not only has the number of advanced heart failure patients risen, but the heart transplant candidates are more complex [5,7]. In spite of the great advances in the field of transplantation, heart transplant professionals and patients still have to face many challenges. Regarding HTx in chagasic patients, the experiences in Brazil in the 1980s established the viability of HTx for Chagas cardiomyopathy as an alternative form of treatment [8,9]. In spite of this, a worldwide spread of Chagas disease and the complexity of reactivation of the *Trypanosoma cruzi* infection have brought major problems to the field. Therefore, more than 50 years later, the differential diagnosis between rejection and *T. cruzi* reactivation poses similar challenges as those faced by Dr. Barnard.

2. The Economic Burden of Chagas Disease

At present, Chagas disease poses a major public health challenge for the Americas, as well as for non-endemic regions around the world, including the United States, Canada, Countries in the European Union, Australia, and Japan [10].

A model for studies of the economic burden of Chagas-disease expansion beyond tropical and sub-tropical zones has been proposed to calculate the healthcare costs and disability-adjusted life-years (DALYs) for individuals, countries, and regions, resulting in an estimate of 7,968,094 infected individuals across the word [10].

For each chronic Chagas disease-infected individual, the calculated cost per year has shown an average cost of USD 383, USD 1762, and USD 2162 in Latin America, Europe, and USA, respectively. The calculated annual cost per person is USD 4660 with a lifetime cost per person of USD 27,684. The global costs per year are estimated to be USD 7,190,000,000, and the cost per lifetime around USD 188.8 billion. This summary of economic burden suggests more attention and effort is needed in the control of Chagas disease [10].

3. Peculiarities of Chagas Disease in the Heart Transplant Setting

Chagas disease infects nearly seven million people in the world, the majority in Latin America [11]. The clinical course of the disease is characterized by an acute phase with patent parasitemia and proliferation of amastigote forms in several tissues. Symptoms subside in a few months and most patients pass to an asymptomatic form of the chronic phase, named the indeterminate phase, with low parasitemia in the blood and tissues. Decades after an initial infection, 20% to 30% of the patients develop chronic cardiopathy, including arrhythmias, conduction defects, sudden cardiac death, and heart failure [12]. The mortality of heart failure patients due to Chagas disease is higher than that observed in other cardiomyopathies [13].

Despite the fact that Chagas disease is a long-life infection, the anti-trypanosomal therapy for infected people during the chronic phase of the disease is not clearly effective and remains a challenge [14].

Heart transplantation is a therapeutic option for those patients with advanced heart failure refractory to medical therapy. Reactivation of Chagas disease is a common finding under immunosuppressive conditions, such as AIDS, autoimmune diseases, cancer (and the chemotherapy used to treat it), and obviously, pharmacological immunosuppression to avoid allograph rejection [7,15].

3.1. Patient Selection

The experience in Brazil in the 1980s established the viability of HTx for Chagas cardiomyopathy as an alternative form of treatment. Currently, HTx is an important therapeutic tool for chagasic patients with advanced heart failure and constitutes the third leading indication for HTx in Brazil [8,9].

The indications and contraindications for HTx follow the classic criteria for other etiologies of heart failure, but some peculiarities are often observed [7,8]. Chagasic patients have lower pulmonary artery pressure, pulmonary vascular resistance, and transpulmonary gradient, which can reduce right ventricular dysfunction, a frequent complication in the post-operative period of HTx [8]. Thus, some transplant centers do not perform cardiac manometry by right cardiac catheterization if the systolic pressure in the pulmonary artery, as estimated by the Doppler-echocardiogram, is <50 mmHg [8]. In general, chagasic patients have a less favorable social and cultural profile, which makes the feasibility of complex procedures such as HTx a challenge. However, there does not seem to be a relationship between the socioeconomic situation and the evolution after HTx [16]. The possibility of megaesophagus and megacolon should be evaluated, which, depending on the severity, may constitute contraindications to HTx [17].

Serology for *T. cruzi* infection in all potential donors and recipients from endemic areas is mandatory, and a donor who tests positive is not accepted for heart recipients. Potential organ donors and recipients should always be screened for the possibility of Chagas disease in endemic countries as well as in non-endemic countries, where the potential donor/recipient ratio has a positive epidemiology [12].

3.2. Immunosuppression Strategies

One of the goals of transplantation science is to equilibrate the immunosuppression, to prevent rejection, and to reduce infection with the occurrence of drug toxicity. Immunosuppressive regimens to prevent rejection can be done by induction (i.e., intense early perioperative/post-operative techniques) and maintenance (i.e., for life) [18–20]. Some categories of recipient candidates (juvenile patients, patients with history of pregnancy or multiple blood transfusions, those on mechanical circulatory support (MCS), and sensitized patients) are supposed to benefit from induction therapy; whereas calcineurin inhibitors, antimetabolite agents, proliferation signal inhibitors, and glucocorticoids are used for maintenance immunosuppression [4].

The main inducing agents are polyclonal anti-thymocyte immunoglobulins (polyclonal antibody—thymoglobulin) and interleukin 2 receptor inhibitors (IL-2), such as daclizumab and basiliximab, which have low immunogenicity [4].

Basic immunosuppressive therapy for the maintenance of cardiac transplant patients in general necessarily includes a calcineurin inhibiting agent, namely, cyclosporin A or tacrolimus. These agents must be associated with mycophenolate mofetil (MMF), mycophenolate sodium, azathioprine, rapamycin, or everolimus. Prednisone is associated with this standard regimen, and in most patients, it can be suspended 6 months after transplantation, in the absence of rejection [4].

In the context of Chagas disease, induction and/or maintenance immunosuppressive therapy can reactivate the *T. cruzi* infection [8,20]. There are no studies comparing the various immunosuppression regimens in chagasic patients, however, a greater number of reactivations have been diagnosed with the use of MMF [21]. Therefore, it would be recommended that chagasic patients receive immunosuppressive therapy with the lowest possible doses, as long as there is no rejection. To prevent rejection-induced reactivation, strategies based on generic principles have been proposed [8]:

1. Reduction in the immunosuppression (which facilitates graft rejection);
2. The use of low doses of several drugs whenever feasible;
3. The avoidance of excessive doses of immunosuppressive agents.

4. Allograph Rejection following Heart Transplantation

Allograft rejection is an important cause of death after heart transplant, in spite of the scientific advances in the field [22–24].

The main types of rejection are as follows: hyperacute, acute cellular (ACR), and antibody-mediated (AMR).

The International Society for Heart and Lung Transplantation (ISHLT) has redefined the pathological diagnosis of both ACR and AMR rejections by grading their severity. ACR is graded as: 0R (no rejection), 1R (mild), 2R (moderate), or 3R (severe). AMR is graded based on immunological (I) or histopathological (p) parameters as follows: pAMR 0 (negative); pAMR1(H+) (p positive and I negative); pAMR1(I+) (p negative and I positive), pAMR2 (both I and p positive), and pAMR3 (severe p) [22,23]. Antibody-mediated rejection has not been frequently reported after HTx in chagasic patients but it can occur [8].

Acute cellular rejection seems to be the predominant type of rejection in such patients. A 70% occurrence of ACR was reported within the first year after HTx, with a 10% mortality rate in chagasic recipients [9,15,25].

The incidence of rejection in chagasic and non-chagasic recipients does not seem to be different [8]. Endomyocardial biopsy, in spite of its invasiveness, is the most used method to monitor and diagnose ACR. Under routine histopathological staining techniques, parasites may not be seen, and the inflammatory infiltrate of rejection (grade 2R or 3R) and reactivation episodes are quite similar; thus, the differential diagnosis between inflammation caused by rejection or reactivation is a difficult task. The protocols for treatment of allograft rejection in both chagasic and non-chagasic recipients are similar. The majority of cases presenting ACR respond properly to pulse corticosteroid therapy, although rescue therapy may be required for selected cases [8].

In addition, a high percentage (up to 43%) of inflammatory infiltrates found to be compatible with the diagnosis of 2R or 3R rejection do not respond to immunosuppressive therapy, but show a good response to antitrypanosomal drugs. Therefore, the detection of an inflammatory mononuclear infiltrate in the endomyocardial biopsy is not enough to rule out the diagnosis of Chagas disease reactivation and poses a challenge, as the most common drug to abort rejection (corticosteroid) may facilitate Chagas disease reactivation. Over 85% of patients have at least one rejection episode before reactivation occurs [8,25].

5. Reactivation

T. cruzi reactivation after HTx is closely related to aggressive immunosuppression. As high immunosuppression protocols induce more frequent Chagas disease reactivation episodes after HTx and affect 20% to 45% of recipients in the first year, an early diagnosis of reactivation is necessarily aimed at pre-emptive therapy. Type I T helper immune response is an important mechanism involved in the *T. cruzi* infection. It is well established that high-dose corticosteroid is able to modify the cytokine profile of type I T helper lymphocytes and is associated with the antiproliferative effect of MMF on T lymphocytes. This environment constitutes a favorable condition for Chagas disease reactivation, which properly treated results in less than 1% mortality. Current evidence indicates that the probability of reactivation could be as high as 90% at 2 years following HTx. Symptoms may be quite similar to those seen in the acute phase of Chagas disease as well as in rejection episodes and include fever, anorexia, myalgia, diarrhea, panniculitis, myocarditis, meningoencephalitis, and encephalic vascular accident [26–29].

Different regimens using immunosuppressive drug associations have not been tested in HTx for chagasic cardiomyopathy. MMF in maintenance immunosuppression seems to be more closely associated with reactivation episodes than the regimens that do not use this drug. Therefore, strategies to change the immunosuppression regimen, such as replacement of MMF by azathioprine or decreasing MMF, have been proposed [21], although no randomized clinical trials are yet available. An early reduction in immunosuppressant agents (especially corticosteroids) is recommended to prevent reactivation, but this approach may facilitate rejection episodes [20,30].

It should be remembered that Chagas disease may affect non-chagasic patients receiving organs from donors with chronic Chagas disease [17,31].

5.1. Reactivation Diagnosis

Reactivation episodes of Chagas disease after HTx have been described as myocarditis, panniculitis, meningoencephalitis, and brain abscess (Figure 1). Myocarditis, the most frequent manifestation, may be asymptomatic or present severe symptoms compatible with heart failure or cardiogenic shock. New skin nodules are characteristic of reactivation. These nodules may ulcerate and the presence of nests of amastigotes is a common skin biopsy finding. Cardiac allograft involvement can manifest as tachycardia, cardiac arrhythmias, A-V blocks, ventricular dysfunction, and cardiogenic shock. Reactivation episodes may induce clinical acute Chagas disease-like symptoms, including fever, anemia, jaundice, liver function test alterations, myocarditis, and neurologic symptoms, secondary to the parasitic effects on the central nervous system. [12,29,32]. However, reactivation episodes may occur without symptoms.

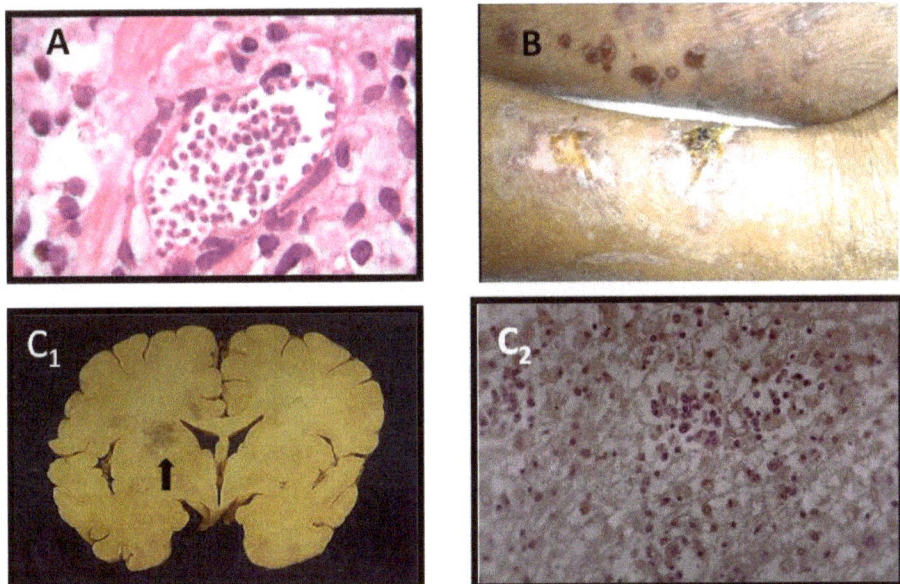

Figure 1. Illustration of Chagas disease reactivation in heart (**A**), skin (**B**), and brain (**C**) in chagasic patients submitted to HTx). (**A**)—Myocarditis in an endomyocardial biopsy showing a nest of amastigotes in the transplanted heart (hematoxylin-eosin staining). (**B**)—Skin lesions in a heart-transplanted chagasic patient. The histology of a biopsied lesion demonstrated a nest of amastigotes (Not shown). (**C**)—Brain lesions in Chagas disease reactivation after heart transplant. (**C1**)—Post-mortem examination showing chagasic encephalitis in a brain macroscopic slice (arrow). (**C2**)—Nests of amastigotes as demonstrated by histopathologic examination (histochemistry: immunoperoxidase technique staining).

Asymptomatic individuals, with tissue or blood samples persistently showing the presence of *T. cruzi* are strong candidates for infection reactivation. The Latin American Guideline for the Diagnosis and Treatment of Chagas Heart Disease has listed some risk factors associated with *T. cruzi* infection reactivation as follows: the number of rejection episodes; the presence of malignancy; immunosuppression grade; use of MMF; autoimmune diseases; HIV infection; and other immunosuppression status [8,30].

The diagnosis of reactivation episodes can be made when symptoms of Chagas disease infection are present. However, diagnosis from only the clinical features is insufficient, i.e., both clinical symptoms and the positive detection of parasites in the blood, cerebrospinal fluid, endomyocardial biopsy, or other tissue samples must coexist. The detection of parasites is made by direct examination of the blood or cerebrospinal fluid, or by biopsies of any infection site which show *T. cruzi* forms under conventional, immunohistochemistry, or immunofluorescence techniques [8].

At present, polymerase chain reaction (PCR) analysis of the blood, endomyocardial biopsy (EMB), or other tissue biopsies are reliable methods to confirm the presence of *T. cruzi* as compared to other techniques. However, EMB is an invasive approach and although being considered a safe procedure, when performed by an experienced operator, complications and sequelae, such as: access site hematoma, right ventricular perforation, chordae tendineae damage, right bundle branch block, arrhythmias, tricuspid regurgitation, may occur. In addition, coronary artery-to-right ventricular fistula, permanent tricuspid valve regurgitation and scarring of the right interventricular septum, compromising the amount of retrieval tissue in future biopsies may occur [33]. One advantage of PCR analysis is that the *T. cruzi* detection precedes the clinical manifestations of reactivation by two or more months. As a consequence, the time required to reach a diagnosis is less than that required by standard parasitological methods. The evolution of the PCR method has led to the appearance of a number of PCR variants. For example, quantitative PCR has a 95.7% sensitivity and a 100% specificity for parasite detection in the acute phase of Chagas disease. Currently, PCR diagnosis is a precious tool which guides physicians as to whether patients should begin receiving anti-parasite drugs or changes in the immunosuppression protocol [26,34,35].

It is well recognized that the isolation of *T. cruzi* from the blood of chagasic recipients (xenodiagnosis, blood culture) is not considered pathognomonic for the diagnosis of Chagas disease reactivation. The same tests may be positive in patients with the chronic form of Chagas disease. In addition, the Strout test is also an alternative for reactivation diagnosis. On the other hand, serological tests are useless for reactivation diagnosis. Their main indication in organ transplantation is when seronegative patients receive organs from seropositive donors, with the most frequently used being ELISA, indirect immunofluorescence (IIF), and indirect hemagglutination (IHA) [8,12,30,35]. A tendency to substitute the immunofluorescence assay (IFA) for a new test, named the trypomastigote excreted–secreted antigens (TESA) immunoblot, in some centers in the U.S.A. has been observed [36].

In countries where Chagas disease is not endemic, failure to identify patients with Chagas disease reactivation constitutes a major medical and social problem, as severe or fatal outcomes may supervene the incapacity to establish a proper diagnosis. [37,38].

The concept of reactivation must, therefore, be redefined as even if no clinical symptoms are evident, reactivation can be diagnosed by an increase in parasitemia, detected either by direct parasitological techniques or by PCR. In this context, a patient may be considered to be presenting reactivation if a current PCR is positive and the previous PCR result was negative. Similarly, if the former test showed lower parasitemia than the current one, the reactivation diagnosis can be accepted [17,34]. Considering that rejection and reactivation may occur several times, that rejection usually precedes reactivation episodes, that symptoms of each condition are similar, and that both conditions may coexist, a differential diagnosis is fundamental for the treatment. Reactivation may then occur several times even if the first episode was properly treated. Despite the possibility of several reactivation episodes in the transplanted heart, no chagasic chronic cardiomyopathy in the recipient has been described [8], and so the role played by *T. cruzi* itself in the infection reactivation is not clear.

There exists an obvious need to monitor for *T. cruzi* reactivation in order to allow the start of specific treatment, mainly in patients without clinical symptoms [29,39]. Chagasic recipients must be followed-up after HTx and monitored for *T. cruzi* infection reactivation, much as they are monitored for rejection, not only routinely but also at any time when the presence of clinical suspicion occurs. Variations in the protocol occur depending on the transplantation center policy. One such policy suggests monitoring for reactivation by histological demonstration of amastigotes at 1, 3, 5, 6, 9, and 12 months after HTx, or whenever the presence of signs or symptoms are present, such as new skin lesions, fever, or overt acute myocarditis [8]. However, no scientific definition about when and how the monitoring protocol should be applied is available. Some centers agree that monitoring for reactivation should take place during the same time that biopsies aiming at allograph rejection detection are done; others prefer monitoring for reactivation every week for 2 months after HTx, then every 2 weeks until the sixth month, and then, once a month from 6 to 12 months [40].

Differential diagnosis between acute cellular rejection and chagasic myocarditis due to reactivation episodes is not an easy task and poses difficulties. The histopathological findings in both conditions are represented by the presence of lymphocytes surrounding the cardiac muscle cells. Slight differences between the morphology of the infiltrate may be seen. Histological diagnosis of reactivation is confirmed if tissue nests of amastigote forms or antigens are detected. The possibility of toxoplasmosis should always be discarded, which makes the use of immunohistochemistry mandatory to establish the diagnosis of reactivation; skin nodule biopsies showing lymphocytes and histiocytes accumulation may be the clue for confirmation of Chagas reactivation. Intense proliferation of *T. cruzi* amastigotes inside macrophages and endothelial cells warrant the diagnosis. However, in the absence of amastigote forms, it is often difficult, even for experienced pathologists, to diagnose the etiology of skin lesions. If parasitic nests of amastigotes are not found in histological sequential sections, the diagnosis of reactivation remains presumptive [18,41]. In the presence of parasitic nests, the way to confirm the etiological nature of the nests is to detect *T. cruzi* antigens by immunohistochemistry. PCR analysis helps a lot in this context. If PCR can distinguish between living and dead trypanosomes after reactivation treatment, it is not known, but certainly parasite DNA and antigen may persist for a period of time in lesions and thus a positive PCR may not always be indicative of an active site of infection [29,41].

Polymerase chain reaction seems to be the topline laboratory method contributing to the diagnosis of reactivation, but both conditions may coexist, and one or more episodes of rejection usually precede the reactivation process. Surveillance for life by a multidisciplinary team is therefore fundamental to the outcome of HTx. The major challenge is to monitor laboratory evidence of Chagas disease reactivation, allowing for etiological treatment before the onset of clinical manifestations, and to prevent severe symptoms and damage to the transplanted heart. [26,34,35,42]

5.2. Results of Heart Transplantation in Chagasic Cardiomyopathy Concerning Reactivation

Evaluation for Chagas reactivation was conducted in 107 adult patients submitted to HTx at InCor, São Paulo, Brazil. The diagnosis of reactivation was accepted only in the case of histological confirmation. In 43 out of the 107 studied patients (40.2%), Chagas reactivation was confirmed. Twenty-three of these 43 patients (53.5%) had the diagnosis confirmed by endomyocardial biopsy, 11 (25.6%) by blood samples testing, 8 (18.6%) by skin, and 1 (2.3%) by brain biopsy. The majority of patients used corticosteroids and MMF. No death or severe graft dysfunction were related to the reactivation episodes [9].

A similar study was conducted in the U.S.A. for Chagas disease after HTx in 31 recipients. Evidence of *T. cruzi* infection reactivation was found in 19 (61%). The median time for reactivation was 3 weeks after HTx (from <1 to 89 weeks). PCR monitoring allowed the diagnosis before manifestation of clinical symptoms in 18 patients, and in only one patient reactivation was diagnosed after the onset of clinical manifestation. No death in this reactivation group was reported after a median of 60 weeks [43].

The HTx in patients with chagasic cardiomyopathy seems to present a better outcome than in non-chagasic recipients. Several factors have been suggested to contribute to this outcome: lower age, less co-morbidities, lower severity grade of rejections, lower incidence of CAV, lower prevalence of pulmonary hypertension, and no history of cardiac surgery before HTx [8,42]. The reported higher incidence of neoplasms after HTx for Chagas disease has not been confirmed in transplanted patients, possibly because of the use of lower doses of immunosuppressive agents, with the aim of avoiding Chagas disease reactivation. The advent of malignancy in HTx of chagasic recipients contributes to death in about 2% of them [8,42–44].

At present, infection and rejection are the major causes of death amongst chagasic recipients of HTx, occurring in 21% and 10–14% of patients, respectively. Cardiac allograft vasculopathy and neoplasms do not seem to be frequent causes of death in HTx chagasic recipients [9].

The native heart may present myocarditis secondary to the presence of *T. cruzi* parasites. This finding does not seem to be associated with Chagas disease reactivation after HTx [8].

5.3. Etiological Treatment of Reactivation

The etiological treatment of Chagas disease is an attractive approach as it could modify the evolution of the disease. Benznidazole and nifurtimox are the anti-trypanosomal drugs of choice, which have been shown to be effective when administered to patients in the acute phase of the disease [12,45]. However, their efficacy on the chronic phase has been a subject of debate [45–48].

Benznidazole seems to be effective in children with *T.cruzi* chronic infection (early chronic phase, less than 15 years), as demonstrated in two placebo-controlled trials, that showed cure rates of approximately 60%, on the basis of conversion to negative serologic test results after treatment [49,50] A large prospective randomized multicenter study on Chagas cardiomyopathy, benznidazole treatment was unable to prevent the cardiac clinical progression although have reduced the parasitemia [51].

The etiological treatment of adults in the indeterminate phase, or very early signs of cardiac involvement, remains unanswered [52,53]. Antiparasitic treatment is not recommended for patients in the chronic phase with advanced Chagas heart disease, as is the case of the heart transplant candidates, since there is no evidence of benefit [12].

The recommendation of benznidazole as a prophylactic agent for all chagasic patients submitted to HTx is questionable due to the lack of available scientific data to support this practice. Besides this, only a percentage of the recipients develop reactivation, and the toxicity and side effects of the drugs might, in some circumstances, be prohibitive. The current recommendation for chagasic HTx is to start anti-trypanosoma treatment whenever Chagas reactivation is confirmed [17,40,41].

Benznidazole and nifurtimox are the trypanocidal drugs of choice, as both compounds are active against trypanosoma. The therapeutic regimens for reactivation are typically made with benznidazole as the first-line drug and nifurtimox as the second option (i.e., for parasite strains resistant to benznidazole) [40–42].

Benznidazole tablets contain 100 mg of active substance. The drug is absorbed in the intestine, processed by the liver cytochrome P-450 system, and excreted predominantly in the urine with a half-life of 12 hours. The recommended posology is 2.5–5 mg·kg^{-1} two times a day (bid). The proposed duration of treatment is 60 days, with a possible extension, depending on the case, to 90 days [51]. The more prominent collateral effect is an urticariform rash, occurring in about 30–60% of patients, usually appearing in the first week of treatment and treated with anti-histamine drugs or with low doses of corticosteroids. If fever and lymph node enlargement appear, benznidazole intake should be interrupted. Less common adverse effects include a late peripheral polyneuropathy manifesting as pain and tingling in the legs, anorexia, insomnia, and bone marrow suppression (which is of rare occurrence), which also imply treatment interruption. Another option is the use of nifurtimox (120 mg/tablet, 8–10 mg/kg), but this medicine is not available in Brazil. The capacity of benznidazole (and nifurtimox) to eliminate the circulating parasites in about 2 weeks and to affect the host immune response is well known, due to its cytotoxic effects on T-cells. These considerations reinforce the importance of benznidazole as a treatment of Chagas disease reactivation [12,30,48].

Both benznidazole or nifurtimox have been contraindicated in pregnant women, as well as in patients with hepatic or renal failure.

It should be reinforced that the same recipient may evolve with more than one episode of Chagas reactivation, needing multiple treatments and increasing the possibility of adverse effects.

6. Heart Transplantation Complications and Survival

The clinical outcome, morbidity, and mortality rates after HTx are similar when chagasic and non-chagasic recipients are compared in the early post-operative period. The major complications after HTx are related to graft dysfunction (20%); rejection (grade 2R or 3R) (10–20%); acute kidney failure (up to 70%) [54]; bleeding (10%); non-*T. cruzi* infection, mainly those located in the respiratory tract (20–30%) [21]. The MCS for chagasic patients with severe cardiomyopathy is not common in Brazil, but when used, no difference in survival was noticed, as compared to patients without bridged MCS [25]. Right ventricular insufficiency, in general, improves with time.

The survival rate of HTx in chagasic patients is better than that for HTx in patients with no Chagas disease. A lower incidence of post-transplant cardiac allograph rejection and a low mortality related to reactivation of Chagas disease have been reported [44]. The actual overall survival of HTx patients with Chagas cardiomyopathy at 1, 5, and 12 years is better than the survival of recipients of HTx with either ischemic or idiopathic cardiomyopathy (the first and second causes of HTx in Brazil, respectively). The survival rates of HTx for Chagas disease have been reported as 76%, 71%, and 46%, at 6 months, 1 year, and 10 years, respectively [21,26,44].

7. Conclusions

Chagas disease (American trypanosomiasis) was originally a health problem endemic to South America, predominantly affecting residents of poor rural areas. The migration of *T. cruzi*-infected individuals to large cities and to developed, non-endemic countries has promoted the worldwide dissemination of Chagas disease. Some of these emigrants are submitted to HTx in the new host non-endemic country, and as a consequence, many reports of reactivation of Chagas disease in HTx patients have been published.

Chagas disease reactivation may occur as a consequence of immunosuppression from several causes, but most published reports of this condition have focused on HTx recipients.

The high number of HTx for chagasic cardiomyopathy in Brazil has meant that there is an accumulation of experience in this field, and thus, has brought the attention of international scientific organizations looking for partnerships to build global recommendations for prevention, early diagnosis, and treatment approaches concerning Chagas disease.

The diagnosis of rejection and/or reactivation in chagasic patients submitted to HTx is not an easy task. PCR seems to be the topline laboratory method, contributing to the differential diagnosis between reactivation and rejection episodes. A complication factor in this issue is the occurrence of one or more episodes of rejection, usually preceding the Chagas disease reactivation process.

Efforts to find laboratory evidence of Chagas disease reactivation, thus allowing therapeutic maneuvers before the onset of clinical manifestations, are intended to prevent severe symptoms and damage to the transplanted heart.

Benznidazole and nifurtimox, in spite of their adverse effects, are the drugs currently eligible for the treatment of Chagas disease reactivation following HTx.

The etiological treatment of HTx recipients without clinical manifestations of Chagas reactivation but showing a positive PCR assay for *T. cruzi* deserve further investigation and a multicenter trial.

Author Contributions: The two authors have worked together and equally contributed to: conceptualization, methodology, formal analysis investigation, writing original draft preparation, writing review and editing. All authors have read and agreed to the published version of the manuscript.

Funding: This research received no external funding.

Acknowledgments: J.R. Cunha-Melo thanks the Brazilian National Council of Research and Scientific Development (CNPq) and Coordenação de Aperfeiçoamento de Pessoal de Nível Superior (CAPES) for scholarships.

Conflicts of Interest: The authors have no conflict of interest to disclose.

References

1. Barnard, C.N. The operation. A human cardiac transplant: An interim report of a successful operation performed at Groote Schuur Hospital, Cape Town. *S. Afr. Med. J.* **1967**, *41*, 1271–1274. [PubMed]
2. Brink, J.G.; Hassoulas, J. The first human heart transplant and further advances in cardiac transplantation at Groote Schuur Hospital and the University of Cape Town. *Cardiovasc. J. Afr.* **2009**, *20*, 31–35. [PubMed]
3. Hunt, S.A.; Haddad, F. The changing face of heart transplantation. *J. Am. Coll. Cardiol.* **2008**, *52*, 587–598. [CrossRef] [PubMed]

4. Khush, K.K.; Cherikh, W.S.; Chambers, D.C.; Harhay, M.O.; Hayes, D.; Hsich, E.; Meiser, B.; Potena, L.; Robinson, A.; Rossano, J.W.; et al. The international thoracic organ transplant registry of the international society for heart and lung transplantation: Thirty-sixth adult heart transplantation report—2019; focus theme: Donor and recipient size match. *J. Heart Lung Transplant.* **2019**, *38*, 1056–1066. [CrossRef] [PubMed]
5. Kobashigawa, J.; Khush, K.; Colvin, M.; Acker, M.; Van Bakel, A.; Eisen, H.; Naka, Y.; Patel, J.; Baran, D.A.; Daun, T.; et al. Report from the american society of transplantation conference on donor heart selection in adult cardiac transplantation in the United States. *Arab. Archaeol. Epigr.* **2017**, *17*, 2559–2566. [CrossRef] [PubMed]
6. Kim, I.-C.; Youn, J.-C.; Kobashigawa, J. The past, present and future of heart transplantation. *Korean Circ. J.* **2018**, *48*, 565–590. [CrossRef] [PubMed]
7. Mehra, M.R.; Canter, C.E.; Hannan, M.M.; Semigran, M.J.; Uber, P.A.; Baran, D.A.; Danziger-Isakov, L.; Kirklin, J.K.; Kirk, R.; Kushwaha, S.S.; et al. The 2016 international society for heart lung transplantation listing criteria for heart transplantation: A 10-year update. *J. Heart Lung Transplant.* **2016**, *35*, 1–23. [CrossRef]
8. Andrade, J.P.; Marin-Neto, J.A.; Paola, A.A.; Vilas-Boas, F.; Oliveira, G.M.; Bacal, F.; Bocchi, E.A.; Almeida, D.R.; Fragata-Filho, A.A.; Moreira, M.C.V.; et al. Sociedade Brasileira de Cardiologia. I Diretriz Latino Americana para o Diagnóstico e Tratamento da Cardiopatia Chagásica. *Arq. Bras. Cardiol.* **2011**, *97*, 1–48. [CrossRef]
9. Fiorelli, A.; Santos, R.; Oliveira, J.L.; Lourenço-Filho, D.; Dias, R.; Oliveira, A.; Da Silva, M.; Ayoub, F.; Bacal, F.; Souza, G.; et al. Heart transplantation in 107 cases of Chagas' disease. *Transplant. Proc.* **2011**, *43*, 220–224. [CrossRef]
10. Lee, B.Y.; Bacon, K.M.; Bottazzi, M.E.; Hotez, P.J. Global economic burden of Chagas disease: A computational simulation model. *Lancet Infect. Dis.* **2013**, *13*, 342–348. [CrossRef]
11. World Health Organization. Chagas Disease (American Trypanosomiaisis [Internet]. Geneva: World Health Organization 2015. Available online: http://www.who.Int/mediacentre/factsheets/fs340/en/ (accessed on 29 May 2020).
12. Dias, J.C.P.; Ramos, A.N.R., Jr.; Gontijo, E.D.; Luquetti, A.; Shikanai-Yasuda, M.A.; Coura, J.R.; Torres, R.M.; Melo, J.R.D.C.; De Almeida, E.A.; Oliveira, W., Jr.; et al. 2nd Brazilian consensus on Chagas disease, 2015. *Rev. Soc. Bras. Med. Trop.* **2016**, *49*, 3–60. [CrossRef] [PubMed]
13. Freitas, H.; Chizzola, P.R.; Paes, Â.; Lima, A.C.; Mansur, A.J. Risk stratification in a Brazilian hospital-based cohort of 1220 outpatients with heart failure: Role of Chagas' heart disease. *Int. J. Cardiol.* **2005**, *102*, 239–247. [CrossRef] [PubMed]
14. Bern, C. A new epoch in antitrypanosomal treatment for Chagas disease. *J. Am. Coll. Cardiol.* **2017**, *69*, 948–950. [CrossRef] [PubMed]
15. Bocchi, E.A.; Fiorelli, A. First guideline group for heart transplantation of the Brazilian Society of Cardiology: The Brazilian experience with heart transplantation: A multicenter report. *J. Heart Lung Transplant.* **2001**, *20*, 637–645. [CrossRef]
16. Parra, A.V.; Rodrigues, V.; Cancella, S.; Cordeiro, J.A.; Bestetti, R.B. Impact of socioeconomic status on outcome of a Brazilian heart transplant recipients cohort. *Int. J. Cardiol.* **2008**, *125*, 142–143. [CrossRef]
17. Pinazo, M.J.; Miranda, B.; Rodríguez-Villar, C.; Altclas, J.; Serra, M.B.; García-Otero, E.C.; De Almeida, E.A.; García, M.M.; Gascon, J.; Rodríguez, M.G.; et al. Recommendations for management of Chagas disease in organ and hematopoietic tissue transplantation programs in nonendemic areas. *Transplant. Rev.* **2011**, *25*, 91–101. [CrossRef]
18. Pinazo, M.J.; Espinosa, G.; Cortes-Lletget, C.; Posada, E.D.J.; Aldasoro, E.; Oliveira, I.; Muñoz, J.; Gállego, M.; Gascon, J. Immunosuppression and Chagas disease: A management challenge. *PLoS Negl. Trop. Dis.* **2013**, *7*. [CrossRef]
19. Costanzo, M.R.; Dipchand, A.; Starling, R.; Anderson, A.S.; Chan, M.; Desai, S.; Fedson, S.; Fisher, P.; Gonzales-Stawinski, G.; Martinelli, L.; et al. The international society of heart and lung transplantation guidelines for the care of heart transplant recipients. *J. Heart Lung Transplant.* **2010**, *29*, 914–956. [CrossRef]
20. Bestetti, R.; Theodoropoulos, T.A. A systematic review of studies on heart transplantation for patients with end-stage Chagas' heart disease. *J. Card. Fail.* **2009**, *15*, 249–255. [CrossRef]
21. Bacal, F.; Silva, C.P.; Bocchi, E.A.; Pires, P.V.; Moreira, L.F.P.; Issa, V.S.; Moreira, S.A.; Cruz, F.D.D.; Strabelli, T.; Stolf, N.A.G.; et al. Mychophenolate mofetil increased Chagas disease reactivation in heart transplanted patients: Comparison between two different protocols. *Arab. Archaeol. Epigr.* **2005**, *5*, 2017–2021. [CrossRef]

22. Colvin, M.M.; Cook, J.L.; Chang, P.; Francis, G.; Hsu, D.; Kiernan, M.S.; Kobashigawa, J.; Lindenfeld, J.; Masri, S.C.; Miller, D.; et al. Antibody-mediated rejection in cardiac transplantation: Emerging knowledge in diagnosis and management: A scientific statement from the American heart association. *Circulation* **2015**, *131*, 1608–1639. [CrossRef] [PubMed]

23. Berry, G.J.; Angelini, A.; Burke, M.M.; Bruneval, P.; Fishbein, M.C.; Hammond, E.; Miller, D.; Neil, D.A.; Revelo, M.P.; Rodriguez, E.R.; et al. The ISHLT working formulation for pathologic diagnosis of antibody-mediated rejection in heart transplantation: Evolution and current status (2005–2011). *J. Heart Lung Transplant.* **2011**, *30*, 601–611. [CrossRef] [PubMed]

24. Berry, G.J.; Burke, M.M.; Andersen, C.; Bruneval, P.; Fedrigo, M.; Fishbein, M.C.; Goddard, M.; Hammond, E.H.; Leone, O.; Marboe, C.; et al. The 2013 international society for heart and lung transplantation working formulation for the standardization of nomenclature in the pathologic diagnosis of antibody-mediated rejection in heart transplantation. *J. Heart Lung Transplant.* **2013**, *32*, 1147–1162. [CrossRef] [PubMed]

25. Benatti, R.D.; Oliveira, G.H.; Bacal, F. Heart transplantation for Chagas cardiomyopathy. *J. Heart Lung Transplant.* **2017**, *36*, 597–603. [CrossRef] [PubMed]

26. Da Costa, P.A.; Segatto, M.; Durso, D.F.; Moreira, W.J.D.C.; Junqueira, L.L.; De Castilho, F.M.; De Andrade, S.A.; Gelape, C.L.; Chiari, E.; Teixeira-Carvalho, A.; et al. Early polymerase chain reaction detection of Chagas disease reactivation in heart transplant patients. *J. Heart Lung Transplant.* **2017**, *36*, 797–805. [CrossRef] [PubMed]

27. Benatti, R.D.; Al-Kindi, S.G.; Bacal, F.; Oliveira, G. Heart transplant outcomes in patients with Chagas cardiomyopathy in the United States. *Clin. Transplant.* **2018**, *32*. [CrossRef]

28. Bacal, F.; Silva, C.P.; Pires, P.V.; Mangini, S.; Fiorelli, A.I.; Stolf, N.G.; Bocchi, E.A. Transplantation for Chagas' disease: An overview of immunosuppression and reactivation in the last two decades. *Clin. Transplant.* **2010**, *24*, E29–E34. [CrossRef]

29. Nogueira, S.S.; Felizardo, A.A.; Caldas, I.S.; Gonçalves, R.V.; Novaes, R.D. Challenges of immunosuppressive and anti trypanosomal drug therapy after heart transplantation in patients with chronic Chagas disease: A systematic review of clinical recommendations. *Transplant. Rev. (Orlando)* **2018**, *33*, 157–167. [CrossRef]

30. Campos, S.V.; Strabelli, T.M.V.; Neto, V.A.; Silva, C.P.; Bacal, F.; Bocchi, E.A.; Stolf, N.A.G. Risk factors for Chagas' disease reactivation after heart transplantation. *J. Heart Lung Transplant.* **2008**, *27*, 597–602. [CrossRef]

31. Kransdorf, E.P.; Zakowski, P.C.; Kobashigawa, J. Chagas disease in solid organ and heart transplantation. *Curr. Opin. Infect. Dis.* **2014**, *27*, 418–424. [CrossRef]

32. Camargos, S.; Moreira, M.C.V.; Portela, D.M.M.C.; Lira, J.P.I.; Modesto, F.V.S.; Menezes, G.M.M.; Moreira, D.R. CNS chagoma—Reactivation in an immunosuppressed patient. *Neurology* **2017**, *88*, 605–606. [CrossRef] [PubMed]

33. From, A.M.; Maleszewski, J.J.; Rihal, C.S. Current status of endomyocardial biopsy. *Mayo Clin. Proc.* **2011**, *86*, 1095–1102. [CrossRef] [PubMed]

34. Diez, M.; Favaloro, L.; Bertolotti, A.; Burgos, J.M.; Vigliano, C.; Lastra, M.P.; Levin, M.J.; Arnedo, A.; Nagel, C.; Schijman, A.G.; et al. Usefulness of PCR strategies for early diagnosis of Chagas' disease reactivation and treatment follow-up in heart transplantation. *Am. J. Transp.* **2007**, *7*, 1633–1640. [CrossRef] [PubMed]

35. Fernandes, C.D.; Tiecher, F.M.; Balbinot, M.M.; Liarte, D.B.; Scholl, D.; Steindel, M.; Romanha, A.J. Efficacy of benznidazol treatment for asymptomatic chagasic patients from state of Rio Grande do Sul evaluated during a three years follow-up. *Memórias Instituto Oswaldo Cruz* **2009**, *104*, 27–32. [CrossRef] [PubMed]

36. Umezawa, E.S.; Nascimento, M.S.; Kesper, N.; Coura, J.R.; Borges-Pereira, J.; Junqueira, A.C.; Camargo, M.E. Immunoblot assay using excreted-secreted antigens of Trypanosoma cruzi in serodiagnosis of congenital, acute, and chronic Chagas' disease. *J. Clin. Microbiol.* **1996**, *34*, 2143–2147. [CrossRef]

37. Jackson, Y.; Dang, T.; Schnetzler, B.; Pascual, M.; Meylan, P. Trypanosoma cruzi fatal reactivation in heart transplant recipient in Switzerland. *J. Heart Lung Transplant.* **2011**, *30*, 484–485. [CrossRef]

38. Gómez-P, C.F.; Mantilla-H, J.C.; Rodriguez-Morales, A.J. Fatal Chagas disease among solid-organ transplant recipients in Colombia. *Open Forum Infect. Dis.* **2014**, *1*. [CrossRef]

39. Chin-Hong, P.V.; Schwartz, B.S.; Bern, C.; Montgomery, S.P.; Kontak, S.; Kubak, B.; Morris, M.I.; Nowicki, M.; Wright, C.; Ison, M.G.; et al. Screening and treatment of Chagas disease in organ transplant recipients in the United States: Recommendations from the Chagas in transplant working group. *Am. J. Transplant.* **2011**, *11*, 672–680. [CrossRef]
40. Schwartz, B.S.; Mawhorter, S.D. Parasitic Infections in Solid Organ Transplantation. *Am. J. Transplant.* **2013**, *13*, 280–303. [CrossRef]
41. Bern, C.; Weller, P.F.; Baron, E.L. Chagas disease in the immunosuppressed host. *Curr. Opin. Infect. Dis.* **2012**, *25*, 450–457. [CrossRef]
42. Theodoropoulos, T.A.; Silva, A.G.; Bestetti, R.B. Eosinophil blood count and anemia are associated with Trypanosoma cruzi infection reactivation in Chagas' heart transplant recipients. *Cardiovasc. Pathol.* **2009**, *19*, 191–192. [CrossRef] [PubMed]
43. Gray, E.B.; La Hoz, R.M.; Green, J.S.; Vikram, H.R.; Benedict, T.; Rivera, H.; Montgomery, S.P. Reactivation of Chagas disease among heart transplant recipients in the United States, 2012–2016. *Transpl. Infect. Dis.* **2018**, *20*. [CrossRef] [PubMed]
44. Bocchi, E.A.; Fiorelli, A. The paradox of survival results after transplantation for cardiomyopathy caused by Trypanosoma cruzi. First guidelines group for heart transplantation of the Brazilian society of cardiology. *Ann. Thorac. Surg.* **2001**, *71*, 1833–1838. [CrossRef]
45. Cançado, J.R. Long term evaluation of etiological treatment of Chagas disease with benznidazole. *Revista Instituto Medicina Tropical São Paulo* **2002**, *44*, 29–37. [CrossRef]
46. Olivera, M.J.; Cucunuba, Z.; Valencia-Hernandez, C.A.; Herazo, R.; Agreda-Rudenko, D.; Florez, C.; Duque, S.; Nicholls, R.S. Risk factors for treatment interruption and severe adverse effects to benznidazole in adult patients with Chagas disease. *PLoS ONE* **2017**, *12*. [CrossRef] [PubMed]
47. Olivera, M.J.; Fory, J.A.; Olivera, A.J. Therapeutic drug monitoring of benznidazole and nifurtimox: A systematic review and quality assessment of published clinical practice guidelines. *Rev. Soc. Bras. Med. Trop.* **2017**, *50*, 748–755. [CrossRef]
48. Bern, C.; Montgomery, S.P.; Herwaldt, B.L.; Rassi, A.; Marin-Neto, J.A.; Dantas, R.O.; Maguire, J.H.; Acquatella, H.; Morillo, C.; Kirchhoff, L.V.; et al. Evaluation and Treatment of Chagas Disease in the United States: A systematic review. *JAMA* **2007**, *298*, 2171–2181. [CrossRef]
49. De Andrade, A.L.S.S.; Zicker, F.; De Oliveira, R.M.; Silva, S.A.E.; Luquetti, A.; Travassos, L.R.; Almeida, I.C.; De Andrade, S.S.; De Andrade, J.G.; Martelli, C.M.; et al. Randomised trial of efficacy of benznidazole in treatment of early Trypanosoma cruzi infection. *Lancet* **1996**, *348*, 1407–1413. [CrossRef]
50. Sosa-Estani, S.; Porcel, B.M.; Segura, E.L.; Yampotis, C.; Ruiz, A.M.; Velazquez, E. Efficacy of chemotherapy with benznidazole in children in the indeterminate phase of Chagas' disease. *Am. J. Trop. Med. Hyg.* **1998**, *59*, 526–529. [CrossRef]
51. Morillo, C.A.; Marin-Neto, J.A.; Avezum, A.; Sosa-Estani, S.; Rosas, F.; Villena, E.; Quiroz, R.; Bonilla, R.; Britto, C.; Guhl, F.; et al. Randomized trial of benznidazole for chronic Chagas' cardiomyopathy. *N. Engl. J. Med.* **2015**, *373*, 1295–1306. [CrossRef]
52. Viotti, R.; Vigliano, C.; Armenti, H.; Segura, E. Treatment of chronic Chagas' disease with benznidazole: Clinical and serologic evolution of patients with long-term follow-up. *Am. Heart J.* **1994**, *127*, 151–162. [CrossRef]
53. Maguire, J.H. Treatment of Chagas' disease—Time is running out. *N. Engl. J. Med.* **2015**, *373*, 1369–1370. [CrossRef] [PubMed]
54. Ortega, A.E.; López, Z.R.D.A.; Pérez, R.H.; Millón, C.F.; Martín, A.D.; Palomo, Y.C.; Gallé, E.L. Kidney failure after heart transplantation. *Transplant. Proc.* **2010**, *42*, 3193–3195. [CrossRef] [PubMed]

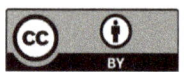

© 2020 by the authors. Licensee MDPI, Basel, Switzerland. This article is an open access article distributed under the terms and conditions of the Creative Commons Attribution (CC BY) license (http://creativecommons.org/licenses/by/4.0/).

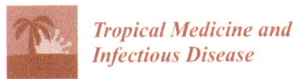

Review

New Imaging Parameters to Predict Sudden Cardiac Death in Chagas Disease

Renata J. Moll-Bernardes [1], Paulo Henrique Rosado-de-Castro [1,2], Gabriel Cordeiro Camargo [1], Fernanda Souza Nogueira Sardinha Mendes [3], Adriana S. X. Brito [1] and Andréa Silvestre Sousa [1,2,3,*]

1. D'Or Institute for Research and Education (IDOR), Rio de Janeiro 22281-100, Brazil; renata.moll@idor.org (R.J.M.-B.); paulo.rosado@idor.org (P.H.R.-d.-C.); gabriel.camargo@idor.org (G.C.C.); adriana.soares@idor.org (A.S.X.B.)
2. Institute of Biomedical Sciences, Federal University of Rio de Janeiro (UFRJ), Rio de Janeiro 21941-901, Brazil
3. Evandro Chagas National Institute of Infectious Diseases, Oswaldo Cruz Foundation, Rio de Janeiro 21040-900, Brazil; fernanda.sardinha@ini.fiocruz.br
* Correspondence: andrea.silvestre@ini.fiocruz.br; Tel.: +55-(21)-999182147

Received: 7 April 2020; Accepted: 6 May 2020; Published: 8 May 2020

Abstract: Chronic Chagas' cardiomyopathy is the most severe and frequent manifestation of Chagas disease, and has a high social and economic burden. New imaging modalities, such as strain echocardiography, nuclear medicine, computed tomography and cardiac magnetic resonance imaging, may detect the presence of myocardial fibrosis, inflammation or sympathetic denervation, three conditions associated with risk of sudden death, providing additional diagnostic and/or prognostic information. Unfortunately, despite its high mortality, there is no clear recommendation for early cardioverter-defibrillator implantation in patients with Chagas heart disease in the current guidelines. Ideally, the risk of sudden cardiac death may be evaluated in earlier stages of the disease using new image methods to allow the implementation of primary preventive strategies.

Keywords: Chagas disease; cardiomyopathy; myocardial fibrosis; myocardial sympathetic denervation; inflammation; sudden death; cardiac magnetic resonance; radionuclide imaging; SPECT-CT; PET-CT

1. Introduction

Chronic Chagas' cardiomyopathy is the most severe and frequent manifestation of Chagas disease and occurs in 25–30% of infected people. Patients may develop severe clinic manifestations, such as congestive heart failure, malignant arrhythmias or thromboembolism [1,2].

The disease is endemic in Latin America, where it is responsible for a high social and economic burden, however, due to the migration of affected individuals and the increased number of patients infected through other forms of transmission, such as blood transfusion, organ transplantation or vertically from mother to infant, the disease has become a global health concern. Non-endemic countries have reported increasing numbers of patients and are particularly worried about the limited awareness in medical community [3]. Cardiac involvement is the main cause of death. The clinical course of Chagas heart disease (CHD) is variable, and the identification of patients at risk for death remains a challenge [4].

The pathogenesis of chronic CHD involves a progressive inflammatory process and adverse immune response with myocardial necrosis and damage to the conduction tissue, leading to electrocardiographic changes, such as atrioventricular and intraventricular blocks, sinus node dysfunction, ventricular arrhythmias and sudden cardiac death. The presence of myocardial inflammation, necrosis and fibrosis may result in left ventricular (LV) segmental wall motion abnormalities and congestive heart failure. Derangements in the coronary microcirculation are likely to cause ischemic-like symptoms, electrocardiographic (ECG) abnormalities and perfusion defects [5].

Patients with CHD are classified according to symptoms and presence of myocardial abnormalities. The presence of typical ECG abnormalities usually defines the diagnosis of chronic CHD (Table 1). The most common initial findings are conduction disorders, and/or ventricular arrhythmias [6].

Table 1. Definition and progression of chronic Chagas heart disease.

Stage	ECG	Echocardiogram	Heart Failure
A	abnormal	Normal	Absent
B1	abnormal	abnormal, LVEF ≥45%	Absent
B2	abnormal	abnormal, LVEF <45%	Absent
C	abnormal	Abnormal	Reversible
D	abnormal	Abnormal	Refractory

Adapted from: Xavier SS et al. [7]. LVEF = left ventricle ejection fraction.

Chronic CHD carries a worse prognosis when compared to ischemic and other non-ischemic causes of heart failure [8]. The presence of chronic persistent myocardial inflammation plays a central role in the genesis of arrhythmias, due to irreversible cell damage, fibrosis and scar formation. Ventricular arrhythmias are a major cause of morbidity and mortality in patients with Chagas disease, and may occur even before significant LV systolic dysfunction, leading to sudden cardiac death (SCD) [9,10]. In addition, active inflammation may increase the automaticity within inflamed areas and act as a trigger for reentry in the presence of fibrosis. Besides fibrosis and inflammation, autonomic dysfunction can also be related to the genesis of ventricular arrhythmias.

Identifying patients with chronic CHD at increased risk of SCD is crucial, as they could benefit from prophylactic implantation of cardioverter-defibrillators [11–13]. ECG, 24 h Holter and exercise test are extremely useful to diagnose and manage these patients. In addition, new imaging modalities such as strain echocardiography, nuclear medicine and cardiac magnetic resonance (CMR) imaging with late gadolinium contrast enhancement may detect the presence of myocardial fibrosis, inflammation or sympathetic denervation, providing additional diagnostic and/or prognostic information. Acute Chagas disease will not be analyzed here.

2. ECG/Holter Monitoring/Exercise Test

2.1. Eletrocardiogram (ECG)

Electrocardiogram (ECG) is the most important exam to characterize in which phase Chagas disease patient is. It is an easy method to perform, widely available worldwide and with high sensitivity. If the ECG remains normal, the prognosis of those patients is similar to the general population. It is important to perform ECG on a serial basis annually to assess possible disease progression. Asymptomatic infected patients with normal ECG (chronic indeterminate form) should be followed annually with clinical evaluation and ECG. In the presence of symptoms and/or ECG abnormalities, patients should be ideally submitted to 24-h Holter, exercise test and echocardiography. Usually, the ECG is the first exam to undergo changes when there is cardiac involvement in the chronic phase of Chagas disease. The presence of typical ECG abnormalities is associated with increased risk of progression to more severe cardiomyopathy.

There are some unspecific findings in ECG that need individualized evaluation, as they alone are not sufficient to diagnose cardiac involvement such as: sinus bradycardia, low voltage QRS, incomplete right bundle branch block, anterosuperior hemiblock, first-degree atrioventricular block and unspecific ST-T findings. The most commons early findings are right bundle branch block with or without left anterior fascicular block, second- and third-degree atrioventricular block. Other alterations associated with CHD are complex ventricular arrythmias, atrial fibrillation, complete atrioventricular block and left brunch block. ECG changes associated with worse prognosis are frequent premature ventricular contractions (PVCs), increased QT-interval dispersion, low-voltage QRS, QRS fragmentation, polymorphous or repetitive non-sustained ventricular tachycardia and prolonged QRS.

When an electrocardiographic alteration compatible with Chagas' disease is identified, the patient is reclassified from chronic undetermined benign form to a cardiac form with a poorer prognosis and additional cardiac and gastrointestinal check-up is recommended (Table 1) [6].

2.2. 24 h Holter

A 24 h Holter is recommended when available and in patients with symptoms suggestive of cardiac arrhythmias, such as palpitations, presyncope and syncope, or ECG abnormalities like bradyarrhythmia, second degree atrioventricular block and multiple PVCs. Often, brady and tachyarrhythmias are identified in the same patient, and this differential diagnosis is important for indicating a pacemaker implant associated or not with the implantable cardioverter defibrillator (ICD). A 24 h Holter is useful to identify an increased risk of sudden cardiac death and unmask signs of autonomic dysfunction, such as reduced heart rate variability. The presence of non-sustained ventricular tachycardia on the 24 h Holter is one criterion that worsens the prognosis of patients with CHD. Major electrocardiographic changes are sinus node dysfunction, atrioventricular block, or frequent PVCs that becomes more complex and frequent with the disease progression. The presence of ventricular tachycardia is associated with left or global ventricular dysfunction and, when sustained, configures a worse prognosis. The main cause of sudden death in CHD is ventricular fibrillation, which is more frequent when there are previous episodes of ventricular tachycardia, but it can be the first manifestation of the disease or its terminal event in patients with severe ventricular dysfunction and heart failure. CHD is one of the most common indications of artificial pacemaker implants in Brazil, and a 24 h Holter is important to help the clinician to confirm the need of the device, indicate the best type and the follow-up after the implant, as this can detect faulty functioning of the stimulation system or orientate better programming [14]. Regarding the autonomic function, a 24 h Holter can assist using spectral analysis. CHD is associated with a reduction in the sympathetic response (reduced LF—low frequency), as well as an overall decrease in autonomic function observed by the reduction of Standard deviation of sequential 5-min N-N interval means (SDANN). The increased rMSSD (square root of the mean of the square of the differences between adjacent normal RR intervals, in a time interval) and pNN50 (percentage of absolute differences in successive normal sinus values >50 ms) values reflect malfunction in their vagal tone.

2.3. Exercise Test

When available, exercise tests should be performed to understand the responses of Chagas disease patients to hemodynamic stress and to assess the functional capacity. The most important finding to observe on ECG during the exam are ventricular arrhythmias, which are independent predictors of mortality [1,15]. They indicate progression of CHD and worsening of cardiomyopathy. The chronotropic response and the heart rate in the first minute of recovery can show how sympathetic and parasympathetic act, since there is an autonomic dysfunction in Chagas disease patients. The assessment of functional capacity is important to guide professional and activity restrictions, to follow the worsening on function capacity and beginning of heart failure. In advanced heart failure patients, the exercise test can suggest a cardiac transplantation indication when the peak oxygen uptake ≤10 mL/kg/min. Finally, exercise test could also useful to access ST changes in differential diagnosis in patients with classical chest pain, to exclude coronary disease and to elucidate patient's symptoms during exercise.

3. Echocardiography

Echocardiography has become the most common method to assess and follow up patients with CHD. The presence of echocardiographic abnormalities allows us to stage disease progression (Table 1). In early stages, echocardiography may demonstrate segmental wall motion abnormalities, particularly in the apex or basal segments of inferior and inferolateral walls, usually without associated obstruction in epicardial coronary arteries [16]. These lesions usually occur due to microcirculatory derangements. Diastolic dysfunction is also a common early finding.

The landmark lesions of CHD are LV apical aneurysms. In order to identify these aneurysms, it is important to use not only standard but also angulated views such as modified four- and two-chambers views, aiming posteriorly and avoiding foreshortening, dropout or near-field artifacts. Aneurysms are not limited to the apex or inferolateral walls, the most common sites, and may be associated to the presence of intraventricular mural thrombi. Right ventricular (RV) aneurysm is uncommon. The prevalence of LV aneurysm is inferior to 10% in asymptomatic patients but has been reported as superior to 50% in patients with more advanced stages, with moderate to severe LV global systolic dysfunction. Symptomatic patients may present regional wall motion abnormalities, LV or biventricular dilatation with diminished LV ejection fraction.

Echocardiograms should be performed at least once in every patient with positive serology and can be repeated each 3–5 years or anytime if ECG abnormalities are detected and should follow the European Association of Cardiovascular Imaging/American Society of Echocardiography task force's recommendations on chamber quantification, LV function and morphology, RV function and valvular analysis [17].

Chamber volumes and global ventricular function should be evaluated by bidimensional (2D) echocardiography through biplane method of disks (Simpson's) and tridimensional (3D) echocardiography, whenever possible. Tridimensional is more accurate than 2D echo for assessing LV volumes and ejection fraction (EF), particularly in the presence of wall motion abnormalities when there is a distorted LV geometry, as it allows visualization of cardiac chambers without geometric assumptions. It can also avoid foreshortening, being more accurate to detect the presence of aneurysms or thrombus. Regional wall motion abnormalities are most often located in the apex, inferior and inferolateral walls and should be assessed in multiple angles. Evaluation should include valvular structure and function, as functional mitral and tricuspid valve regurgitation are common in advanced cases with ventricular remodeling and valve annular dilation.

Strain is a measure of myocardial deformation, defined as the change of length of the myocardium that allows a more precise and quantitative measurement of the regional myocardial function, overcoming the subjective evaluation by conventional echocardiography. Strain obtained by speckle-tracking is the method of choice because it is not angle dependent. Regional strain is of particular interest in CHD due to the frequent segmental myocardial involvement (Figure 1), being particularly useful for increased recognition of subclinical myocardial dysfunction during indeterminate form of CHD [18,19]. Global longitudinal strain is the most validated method and is correlated with the amount of myocardial fibrosis, as shown is a study including 125 patients with Chagas disease, which found that longitudinal strain was reduced in the patients who had cardiac fibrosis on CMR, despite no significant difference in LV ejection fraction compared with patients without cardiac fibrosis [20].

Echocardiography may potentially be used to study ventricular dyssynchrony in CHD [21,22]. Duarte et al. [22] reported that the prevalence of interventricular dyssynchrony was 34% and of intraventricular dyssynchrony was 85%. However, dyssynchrony was not a strong predictor of clinical events, and the ECG remains the most important tool for indicating cardiac resynchronization therapy. Contrast echocardiography can be useful to enhance LV endocardial border and increase detection of aneurysms and thrombus [15].

Echocardiography is an inexpensive and readily available method, being very useful to stage and follow these patients, giving hemodynamic information that can be extremely helpful in advanced heart failure. On the other hand, the method is less sensitive to evaluate the presence of fibrosis and is not able to detect inflammation.

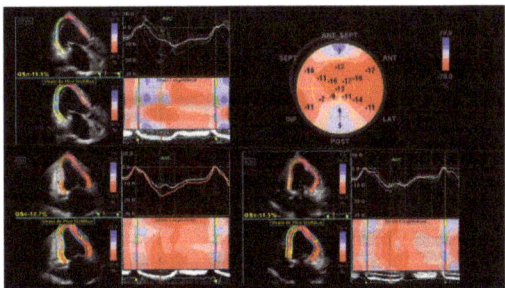

Figure 1. Global longitudinal strain of the left ventricle and strain curves depicting increased mechanical dispersion. Abnormal findings of left ventricular (LV) longitudinal strain in apical three-chamber view (**top left**); apical two-chamber view (**bottom left**); apical four-chamber view (**bottom right**); "Bull's-eye" plot of strain values for each myocardial segment evidences anteroseptal and inferolateral akinesia represented by blue areas in the polar map (**top right**).

4. Computed Tomography

Cardiac computed tomography (CT) has an excellent negative predictive value to exclude coronary artery disease through coronary computed tomography angiogram (CTA), being extremely useful in patients with low to intermediate pre-test probability. Cardiac CT can also be used to plan electrophysiologic procedures, evaluate LV morphology, including the detection of regional wall motion abnormalities, apical aneurysms and intracardiac thrombi, and to calculate LV function in patients with difficult echocardiographic windows and contraindication to CMR, such as the presence of an implanted cardiac device [1,5].

5. Cardiovascular Magnetic Resonance

CMR has a superior capability for anatomic and functional evaluation of cardiac chambers and measurement of right and left ventricular EF. LV systolic dysfunction is the strongest predictor of morbidity and mortality in CHD, and detection of subclinical dysfunction may orient therapeutic measures that would help in delaying the progression of the disease. Regional wall motion abnormalities, thrombus and aneurysms can be easily recognized (Figure 2).

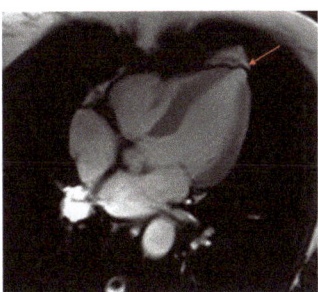

Figure 2. Cardiac magnetic resonance (CMR) four chamber image showing a typical left ventricular mamillar apical aneurysm (arrow). CMR: cardiac magnetic resonance.

Myocardial fibrosis is a histopathological finding common to several types of cardiovascular diseases and is associated with morbidity and mortality [23,24]. The mechanisms leading to fibrosis are variable and there may be an imbalance between collagen production and degradation or myocyte death [25].

The presence of fibrotic myocardial lesions is associated to reentrant circuits, which are the main pathophysiologic mechanism of ventricular tachyarrhythmias. Recent studies reveal that the degree of myocardial fibrosis increases progressively from the mildest to the most severe disease stages and late gadolinium contrast enhancement (LGE) evaluated on CMR is currently the best non-invasive method to assess it, being a marker of subclinical involvement with proven prognostic value [26–28]. The presence of scar by LGE is strongly associated with high risk of SCD [29].

Development of fibrosis in Chagas disease patients predominates in territories of distal circulation, particularly in apical and inferolateral regions, and the pattern of LGE is usually meso-epicardial or transmural (Figure 3), which differs from ischemic cardiomyopathies, in which LGE with a characteristic subendocardial fibrosis pattern matches a coronary territory distribution [11].

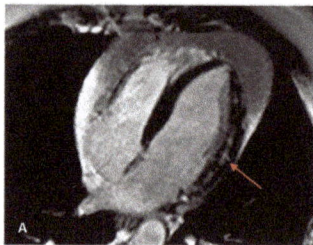 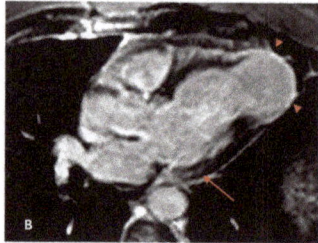

Figure 3. CMR images in four chamber (**A**) and three chamber (**B**) views showing meso-epicardial (arrows) and apical transmural (arrowheads) late gadolinium enhancement (LGE). CMR: cardiac magnetic resonance; LGE: late gadolinium enhancement.

Nonetheless, LGE fails to account for interstitial and diffuse collagen distribution, which leads to underestimation of the total myocardial fibrosis mass [30]. The capability of tissue characterization with detection of myocardial edema and interstitial fibrosis has been recently reported in ischemic and non-ischemic cardiomyopathies and may be helpful in risk assessment [31]. New CMR techniques, such as native T1 mapping (Figure 4) and myocardial extracellular volume (ECV) calculation quantify diffuse myocardial fibrosis with close correlation with histological studies [32]. Avanesov et al. [31] reported that global ECV was superior to other CMR parameters, including LGE, to identify hypertrophic cardiomyopathy patients with syncope and non-sustained ventricular tachycardia, and presumably with increased risk of SCD. Future studies are necessary to evaluate the usefulness of these techniques in Chagas disease.

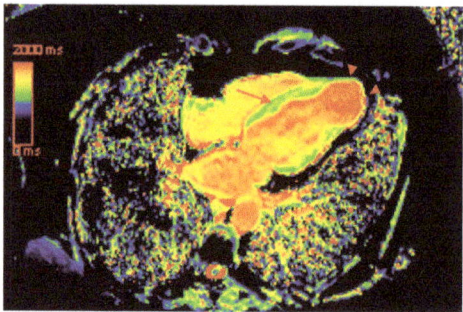

Figure 4. Four chamber image with color-coded native (non-contrast) T1 map, indicating the presence of mesocardial septal fibrosis (arrow) and apical transmural fibrosis (arrowheads). Increased native T1 is represented by yellow areas within the myocardium.

6. Nuclear Medicine

Patients with chronic CHD have an increased risk of SCD compared to other cardiomyopathies. The presence of fibrosis, dysautonomia and persistent cardiac inflammation could contribute to the risk of SCD, offering a substrate for ventricular tachycardia (VT). Molecular imaging with single photon emission computed tomography (SPECT) or positron emission tomography (PET) using a variety of radiotracers are valuable tools to identify changes that predispose to arrhythmia, such as hypoperfusion, inflammation and abnormal sympathetic innervation.

Myocardial perfusion imaging may be performed with SPECT or hybrid SPECT-CT equipment, using technetium-99m labeled radiopharmaceuticals such as tetrofosmin or sestamibi (Figure 5), or with PET and hybrid PET-CT using radiopharmaceuticals such as Rubidium-82. A disturbance due to microvascular ischemia participates in the mechanisms, causing myocardial injury and can occur in the early stages of CHD [33]. The use of hybrid SPECT-CT and PET-CT equipment allows attenuation correction, reducing artifacts.

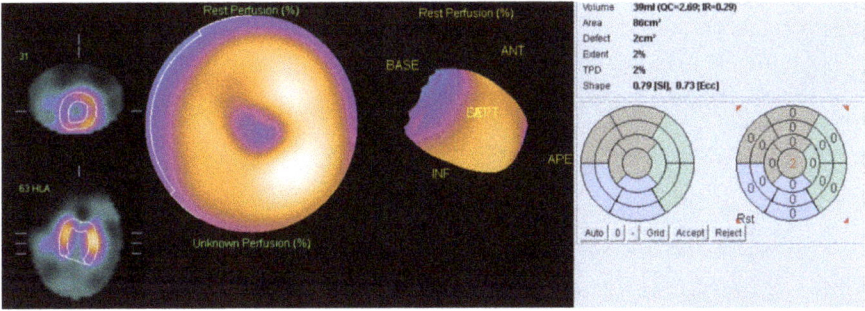

Figure 5. Automatic quantification (polar map) from rest 99m-Technetium sestamibi scintigraphy demonstrating reduced myocardial perfusion in apical region in a patient with a small aneurism of the left ventricular apex.

It has been demonstrated that histogram bandwidth and phase-derived standard deviation may be analyzed in gated-SPECT myocardial perfusion imaging (Figure 6), which allows the assessment of intraventricular synchronism. In comparison to echocardiography, nuclear medicine techniques have the advantage of lower interobserver variability and higher reproducibility. Peix et al. [34] studied myocardial perfusion and intraventricular synchronism in the indeterminate phase of Chagas disease which presented tissue Doppler imaging-derived strain. A total of 8% of subjects had perfusion defects, 28% had a post-stress LVEF reduction of >5%. The authors found that histogram bandwidth and phase-derived standard deviation indicated a significant difference between post-stress and rest. In these cases, there was a minor dyssynchrony at rest that normalized at post-stress.

Abnormalities in cardiac sympathetic innervation may play a central role in the mechanism triggering serious ventricular arrhythmias and SCD in patients with non-ischemic cardiomyopathy. The work of Miranda [35] showed that regional myocardial sympathetic denervation assessed with Iodine-123 metaiodobenzylguanidine (123I-MIBG) scintigraphy is associated with sustained ventricular tachycardia in CHD, concluding that viable although denervated myocardial areas were associated to the genesis of sustained ventricular arrhythmias (Figure 7). Cardiac autonomic sympathetic modulation detected with 123I-MIBG SPECT can also be affected in subjects with early forms of CHD with preserved ventricular function, as reported by Landesmann [36]. Recently, Gadioli [37] used 123I-MIBG SPECT to assess the extension of the sympathetic denervation, and showed its association with the severity of the ventricular arrhythmias. It is necessary to design prospective studies for the assessment of cardiac sympathetic innervation. Results could be used for risk stratifications of sudden death, which would be extremely useful if we consider the lack of consensus related to the stratification and primary prevention of sudden cardiac death in patients with Chagas disease.

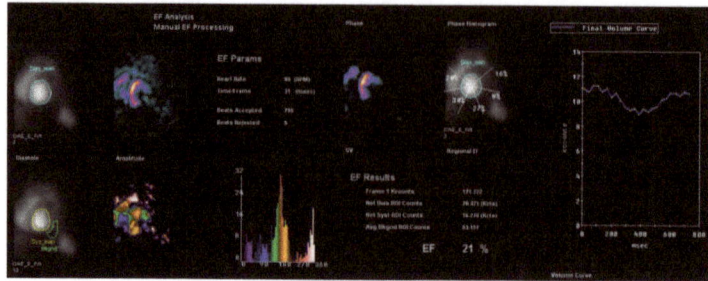

Figure 6. Multigated acquisition (MUGA) scan demonstrating reduced ejection fraction (EF = 21%) in a patient with Chagasic cardiomyopathy. This radionuclide ventriculography technique is a highly accurate test, used to determine the heart's pumping function, and it shows substantial reproducibility and low intraobserver and interobserver variability.

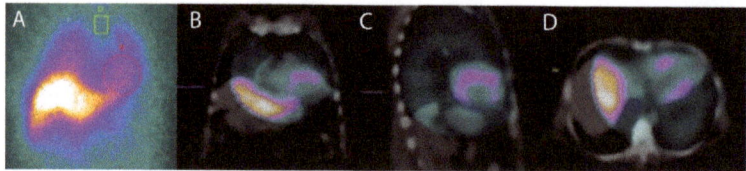

Figure 7. A 123I-MIBG scintigraphy planar scintigraphy in anterior view at 3 h (**A**) to evaluate the sympathetic innervation a patient with Chagasic cardiomyopathy and ventricular arrhythmia. Heart to mediastinum ratio at 3 h was reduced and radiotracer washout was increased. Single photon emission computed tomography (SPECT)-computed tomography (CT) images in coronal (**B**), sagittal (**C**) and transversal (**D**) planes demonstrated reduced cardiac uptake of 123I-MIBG in apical, inferior and lateral regions indicating sympathetic denervation in these areas and a worse prognosis.

The presence of persistent cardiac inflammation may also be related to ventricular tachycardia and the risk of sudden death. Persistent subclinical inflammation in areas adjacent to fibrotic regions may act as a trigger for reentry in the presence of fibrosis. In addition, active inflammation may increase the automaticity within inflamed areas. Radionuclide imaging can allow the identification of areas of inflammation of the myocardium in patients with non-ischemic cardiomyopathies [38].

^{18}F-fluorodeoxyglucose (^{18}F-FDG) is a glucose analogue being physiologically captured by cardiomyocytes which can be used to evaluate the pathologic uptake by inflammatory cells. Recently, the use of ^{18}F-FDG PET-CT has been studied in patients with sarcoidosis, demonstrating that the presence of focal perfusion defects and increased FDG uptake in patients with suspected cardiac sarcoidosis identified subjects at higher risk of death or ventricular tachycardia [39].

The use of PET-CT in Chagas disease has not yet been systematically studied. There are several similarities between Chagas disease and sarcoidosis, so the use of this imaging technique could potentially be useful in assessing the presence of inflammation and prognosis. Both are associated with changes in the conduction system and complex ventricular arrhythmias and with the presence of meso-epicardial fibrosis.

Currently, patients with chronic Chagas disease are not routinely evaluated for the presence of inflammation. Three case reports have described increased uptake of 18F-FDG PET in patients with Chagas disease and ventricular tachycardia, suggesting that the presence of inflammation could be involved in the genesis of the arrhythmia [40,41]. Recently, the use of new radiotracers that are not physiologically accumulated in the normal myocardium, including somatostatin receptor imaging radiopharmaceuticals such as gallium-68 (^{68}Ga) labeled-DOTATOC may overcome some limitations of the ^{18}F-FDG, as has been reported for cardiac sarcoidosis and CHD [42,43], as illustrated in Figure 8.

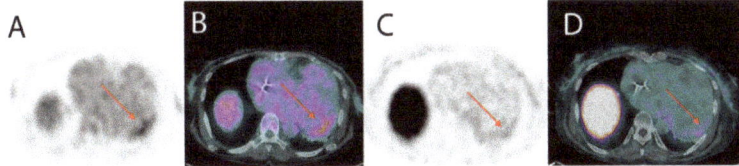

Figure 8. Increased cardiac volume in a patient with Chagasic cardiomyopathy. Mild increase in uptake of 18F-FDG (**A,B**) and of 68Ga-DOTATOC (**C,D**) in positron emission tomography (PET)-CT images was restricted to the basal anterolateral segment, indicating the presence of inflammation in this segment.

PET-CT has the advantage of a higher spatial resolution when compared to scintigraphy and, unlike CMR, it can be used in patients with implantable cardiac devices. Better understanding of the role of inflammation in these patients may provide novel treatment strategies, such as localization of the anatomic substrate before ablation of VT, and improved risk stratification and orientation about primary prevention with ICD implantation.

Unfortunately, despite its significant mortality, there is no clear recommendation for early ICD implantation in patients with CHD in the current guidelines. Ideally, the risk of SCD should be evaluated in earlier stages of the disease. New imaging parameters that are useful to identify factors involved in the genesis of arrhythmia such as fibrosis, inflammation and dysautonomia (Figure 9) can be a promising strategy.

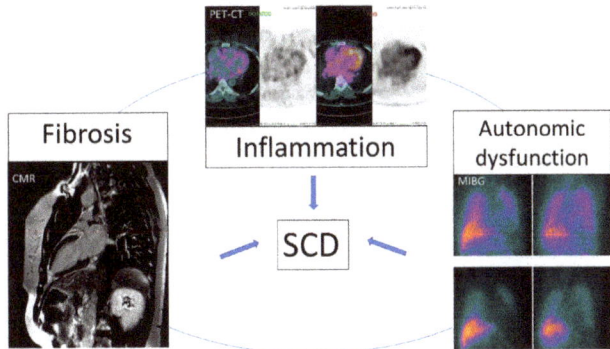

Figure 9. New imaging modalities can detect abnormalities involved in the genesis of ventricular arrythmia. SCD: Sudden cardiac death.

7. Conclusions

Fibrosis, inflammation and dysautonomia are involved in the genesis of ventricular arrhythmia in CHD. Due to the risk of sudden death, it is important that such events are early identified, so that SCD preventive measures can be taken. Myocardial fibrotic areas leads to a macro reentry circuit that triggers ventricular tachycardia and CMR is an accurate method to identify these areas. The presence of inflammatory process, detected through PET-CT with FDG or DOTATOC, may be involved in the genesis of the arrhythmia in CHD. Finally, studies of myocardial dysautonomia identified using myocardial SPECT-CT with MIBG have reported an association between denervated areas and ventricular electrical instability, even in the presence of viable myocardium. Echocardiography, despite not being sensitive enough to identify fibrosis and denervation, can indicate severe ventricular dysfunction, which is also associated with an increased risk of sudden death. Other non-invasive tests such as ECG, 24 h Holter and exercise test can identify both dysautonomia, and the presence of ventricular electrical instability, demonstrating an increased risk of sudden death in CHD patients. Thereby, traditional non-invasive diagnostic methods associated to new image parameters obtained through CMR, SPECT-CT and PET-CT can improve risk stratification of SCD and play a promising role in the implementation of primary preventive strategies.

Funding: This research received no external funding.

Conflicts of Interest: The authors declare no conflict of interest.

References

1. Nunes, M.C.P.; Beaton, A.; Acquatella, H.; Bern, C.; Bolger, A.F.; Echeverria, L.E.; Dutra, W.O.; Gascon, J.; Morillo, C.A.; Oliveira-Filho, J.; et al. Chagas Cardiomyopathy: An Update of Current Clinical Knowledge and Management: A Scientific Statement from the American Heart Association. *Circulation* **2018**, *138*, e169–e209. [CrossRef] [PubMed]
2. De Carvalho Filho, H.A.; de Sousa, A.S.; de Holanda, M.T.; Haffner, P.M.A.; Atié, J.; do Brasil, P.E.A.A.; Hasslocher-Moreno, A.; Xavier, S.S. Valor prognóstico independente da taquicardia ventricular não-sustentada na fase crônica da Doença de Chagas. *Rev. SOCERJ* **2007**, *20*, 395–405.
3. Andrade, J.; Marin-Neto, J.; Paola, A.; Vilas-Boas, F.; Oliveira, G.; Bacal, F.; Bocchi, E.; Almeida, D.; Fragata, F.A.; Moreira, M.C. I Latin American guidelines for the diagnosis and treatment of Chagas cardiomyopathy. *Arq. Bras. Cardiol.* **2011**, *97*, 1. [PubMed]
4. Rassi, A., Jr.; Rassi, A.; Little, W.C.; Xavier, S.S.; Rassi, S.G.; Rassi, A.G.; Rassi, G.G.; Hasslocher-Moreno, A.; Sousa, A.S.; Scanavacca, M.I. Development and validation of a risk score for predicting death in Chagas' heart disease. *N. Engl. J. Med.* **2006**, *355*, 799–808. [CrossRef]
5. Acquatella, H.; Asch, F.M.; Barbosa, M.M.; Barros, M.; Bern, C.; Cavalcante, J.L.; Echeverria Correa, L.E.; Lima, J.; Marcus, R.; Marin-Neto, J.A.; et al. Recommendations for Multimodality Cardiac Imaging in Patients with Chagas Disease: A Report from the American Society of Echocardiography in Collaboration with the InterAmerican Association of Echocardiography (ECOSIAC) and the Cardiovascular Imaging Department of the Brazilian Society of Cardiology (DIC-SBC). *J. Am. Soc. Echocardiogr.* **2018**, *31*, 3–25.
6. Dias, J.C.; Ramos, A.N., Jr.; Gontijo, E.D.; Luquetti, A.; Shikanai-Yasuda, M.A.; Coura, J.R.; Torres, R.M.; Melo, J.R.; Almeida, E.A.; Oliveira, W., Jr.; et al. Brazilian Consensus on Chagas Disease, 2015. *Epidemiol. Serv. Saude* **2016**, *25*, 7–86. [CrossRef]
7. Xavier, S.; Sousa, A.; Hasslocher-Moreno, A. Application of the new classification of cardiac insufficiency (ACC/AHA) in chronic Chagas cardiopathy: A critical analysis of the survival curves. *Rev. SOCERJ* **2005**, *18*, 227–232.
8. Shen, L.; Ramires, F.; Martinez, F.; Bodanese, L.C.; Echeverría, L.E.; Gómez, E.A.; Abraham, W.T.; Dickstein, K.; Køber, L.; Packer, M. Contemporary characteristics and outcomes in chagasic heart failure compared with other nonischemic and ischemic cardiomyopathy. *Circ. Heart Fail.* **2017**, *10*, e004361. [CrossRef]
9. De Souza, A.C.J.; Salles, G.; Hasslocher-Moreno, A.M.; de Sousa, A.S.; do Brasil, P.E.A.A.; Saraiva, R.M.; Xavier, S.S. Development of a risk score to predict sudden death in patients with Chaga's heart disease. *Int. J. Cardiol.* **2015**, *187*, 700–704. [CrossRef]
10. Sternick, E.B.; Martinelli, M.; Sampaio, R.C.; Gerken, L.M.; Teixeira, R.A.; Scarpelli, R.; Scanavacca, M.; Nishioka, S.D.O.; Sosa, E. Sudden cardiac death in patients with chagas heart disease and preserved left ventricular function. *J. Cardiovasc. Electrophysiol.* **2006**, *17*, 113–116. [CrossRef]
11. Moll-Bernardes, R.J.; Saraiva, R.M.; Sarmento de Oliveira, R.; Tavares Pinheiro, M.V.; Camargo, G.C.; Xavier de Brito, A.S.; Altino de Almeida, S.; Siqueira, F.P.; de Souza Nogueira Sardinha Mendes, F.; Barbosa, R.M. Case Report: Malignant Ventricular Arrhythmias Mimicking Acute Coronary Syndrome in Chagas Disease. *Am. J. Trop. Med. Hyg.* **2020**, *102*, 797–799. [CrossRef]
12. Bestetti, R.B.; Dalbo, C.M.; Arruda, C.A.; Correia Filho, D.; Freitas, O.C. Predictors of sudden cardiac death for patients with Chagas' disease: A hospital-derived cohort study. *Cardiology* **1996**, *87*, 481–487. [CrossRef] [PubMed]

13. Bestetti, R.B.; Cardinalli-Neto, A. Sudden cardiac death in Chagas' heart disease in the contemporary era. *Int. J. Cardiol.* **2008**, *131*, 9–17. [CrossRef] [PubMed]
14. Menezes, A., Jr.; Queiroz, C.; Carzola, F.; Dourado, J.; Carvalho, W. Variabilidade da freqüência cardíaca em pacientes com doença de Chagas. *J. Card. Arrhythm.* **2000**, *13*, 139–142.
15. Nunes, M.C.P.; Badano, L.P.; Marin-Neto, J.A.; Edvardsen, T.; Fernandez-Golfin, C.; Bucciarelli-Ducci, C.; Popescu, B.A.; Underwood, R.; Habib, G.; Zamorano, J.L.; et al. Multimodality imaging evaluation of Chagas disease: An expert consensus of Brazilian Cardiovascular Imaging Department (DIC) and the European Association of Cardiovascular Imaging (EACVI). *Eur. Heart J. Cardiovasc. Imaging* **2018**, *19*, 459–460n. [CrossRef] [PubMed]
16. Acquatella, H.; Schiller, N.B.; Puigbó, J.; Giordano, H.; Suárez, J.; Casal, H.; Arreaza, N.; Valecillos, R.; Hirschhaut, E. M-mode and two-dimensional echocardiography in chronic Chages' heart disease. A clinical and pathologic study. *Circulation* **1980**, *62*, 787–799. [CrossRef]
17. Mitchell, C.; Rahko, P.S.; Blauwet, L.A.; Canaday, B.; Finstuen, J.A.; Foster, M.C.; Horton, K.; Ogunyankin, K.O.; Palma, R.A.; Velazquez, E.J. Guidelines for performing a comprehensive transthoracic echocardiographic examination in adults: Recommendations from the American Society of Echocardiography. *J. Am. Soc. Echocardiogr.* **2019**, *32*, 1–64. [CrossRef]
18. Barbosa, M.M.; Rocha, M.O.C.; Vidigal, D.F.; de Carvalho Bicalho Carneiro, R.; Araújo, R.D.; Palma, M.C.; de Barros, M.V.L.; Nunes, M.C.P. Early detection of left ventricular contractility abnormalities by two-dimensional speckle tracking strain in Chagas' disease. *Echocardiography* **2014**, *31*, 623–630. [CrossRef]
19. García-Álvarez, A.; Sitges, M.; Regueiro, A.; Poyatos, S.; Pinazo, M.J.; Posada, E.; Bijnens, B.; Heras, M.; Gascon, J.; Sanz, G. Myocardial deformation analysis in Chagas heart disease with the use of speckle tracking echocardiography. *J. Card. Fail.* **2011**, *17*, 1028–1034. [CrossRef]
20. Gomes, V.A.; Alves, G.F.; Hadlich, M.; Azevedo, C.F.; Pereira, I.M.; Santos, C.R.; Brasil, P.E.; Sangenis, L.H.; Cunha, A.B.; Xavier, S.S.; et al. Analysis of Regional Left Ventricular Strain in Patients with Chagas Disease and Normal Left Ventricular Systolic Function. *J. Am. Soc. Echocardiogr.* **2016**, *29*, 679–688. [CrossRef]
21. Silva Júnior, O.D.; Maeda, P.M.; Borges, M.C.C.; Melo, C.S.D.; Correia, D. One-year cardiac morphological and functional evolution following permanent pacemaker implantation in right ventricular septal position in chagasic patients. *Rev. Soc. Bras. Med. Trop.* **2012**, *45*, 340–345. [CrossRef] [PubMed]
22. Duarte, J.D.O.; Magalhães, L.P.D.; Santana, O.O.; Silva, L.B.D.; Simões, M.; Azevedo, D.O.D. Prevalence and prognostic value of ventricular dyssynchrony in Chagas cardiomyopathy. *Arq. Bras. Cardiol.* **2011**, *96*, 300–306. [CrossRef] [PubMed]
23. Di Marco, A.; Anguera, I.; Schmitt, M.; Klem, I.; Neilan, T.G.; White, J.A.; Sramko, M.; Masci, P.G.; Barison, A.; McKenna, P.; et al. Late Gadolinium Enhancement and the Risk for Ventricular Arrhythmias or Sudden Death in Dilated Cardiomyopathy: Systematic Review and Meta-Analysis. *JACC Heart Fail.* **2017**, *5*, 28–38. [CrossRef] [PubMed]
24. Kwon, D.H.; Halley, C.M.; Carrigan, T.P.; Zysek, V.; Popovic, Z.B.; Setser, R.; Schoenhagen, P.; Starling, R.C.; Flamm, S.D.; Desai, M.Y. Extent of left ventricular scar predicts outcomes in ischemic cardiomyopathy patients with significantly reduced systolic function: A delayed hyperenhancement cardiac magnetic resonance study. *JACC Cardiovasc. Imaging* **2009**, *2*, 34–44. [CrossRef] [PubMed]
25. Rathod, R.H.; Powell, A.J.; Geva, T. Myocardial Fibrosis in Congenital Heart Disease. *Circ. J.* **2016**, *80*, 1300–1307. [CrossRef]
26. Senra, T.; Ianni, B.M.; Costa, A.C.; Mady, C.; Martinelli-Filho, M.; Kalil-Filho, R.; Rochitte, C.E. Long-term prognostic value of myocardial fibrosis in patients with chagas cardiomyopathy. *J. Am. Coll. Cardiol.* **2018**, *72*, 2577–2587. [CrossRef]
27. Regueiro, A.; García-Álvarez, A.; Sitges, M.; Ortiz-Pérez, J.T.; De Caralt, M.T.; Pinazo, M.J.; Posada, E.; Heras, M.; Gascón, J.; Sanz, G. Myocardial involvement in Chagas disease: Insights from cardiac magnetic resonance. *Int. J. Cardiol.* **2013**, *165*, 107–112. [CrossRef]
28. Mello, R.P.D.; Szarf, G.; Schvartzman, P.R.; Nakano, E.M.; Espinosa, M.M.; Szejnfeld, D.; Fernandes, V.; Lima, J.A.; Cirenza, C.; De Paola, A.A. Delayed enhancement cardiac magnetic resonance imaging can identify the risk for ventricular tachycardia in chronic Chagas' heart disease. *Arq. Bras. Cardiol.* **2012**, *98*, 421–430. [CrossRef]

29. Volpe, G.J.; Moreira, H.T.; Trad, H.S.; Wu, K.C.; Braggion-Santos, M.F.; Santos, M.K.; Maciel, B.C.; Pazin-Filho, A.; Marin-Neto, J.A.; Lima, J.A. Left ventricular scar and prognosis in chronic chagas cardiomyopathy. *J. Am. Coll. Cardiol.* **2018**, *72*, 2567–2576. [CrossRef]
30. Torreão, J.A.; Ianni, B.M.; Mady, C.; Naia, E.; Rassi, C.H.; Nomura, C.; Parga, J.R.; Avila, L.F.; Ramires, J.A.; Kalil-Filho, R. Myocardial tissue characterization in Chagas' heart disease by cardiovascular magnetic resonance. *J. Cardiovasc. Magn. Reson.* **2015**, *17*, 97. [CrossRef]
31. Avanesov, M.; Münch, J.; Weinrich, J.; Well, L.; Säring, D.; Stehning, C.; Tahir, E.; Bohnen, S.; Radunski, U.K.; Muellerleile, K. Prediction of the estimated 5-year risk of sudden cardiac death and syncope or non-sustained ventricular tachycardia in patients with hypertrophic cardiomyopathy using late gadolinium enhancement and extracellular volume CMR. *Eur. Radiol.* **2017**, *27*, 5136–5145. [CrossRef] [PubMed]
32. Kammerlander, A.A.; Marzluf, B.A.; Zotter-Tufaro, C.; Aschauer, S.; Duca, F.; Bachmann, A.; Knechtelsdorfer, K.; Wiesinger, M.; Pfaffenberger, S.; Greiser, A. T1 mapping by CMR imaging: From histological validation to clinical implication. *JACC Cardiovasc. Imaging* **2016**, *9*, 14–23. [CrossRef] [PubMed]
33. Simões, M.V.; Pintya, A.O.; Bromberg-Marin, G.; Sarabanda, Á.V.; Antloga, C.M.; Pazin-Filho, A.; Maciel, B.C.; Marin-Neto, J.A. Relation of regional sympathetic denervation and myocardial perfusion disturbance to wall motion impairment in Chagas' cardiomyopathy. *Am. J. Cardiol.* **2000**, *86*, 975–981. [CrossRef]
34. Peix, A.; Garcia, R.; Sanchez, J.; Cabrera, L.O.; Padron, K.; Vedia, O.; Choque, H.V.; Fraga, J.; Bandera, J.; Hernandez-Canero, A. Myocardial perfusion imaging and cardiac involvement in the indeterminate phase of Chagas disease. *Arq. Bras. Cardiol.* **2013**, *100*, 114–117. [CrossRef]
35. Miranda, C.H.; Figueiredo, A.B.; Maciel, B.C.; Marin-Neto, J.A.; Simoes, M.V. Sustained ventricular tachycardia is associated with regional myocardial sympathetic denervation assessed with 123I-metaiodobenzylguanidine in chronic Chagas cardiomyopathy. *J. Nucl. Med.* **2011**, *52*, 504–510. [CrossRef]
36. Landesmann, M.C.P.; da Fonseca, L.M.B.; Pereira, B.D.B.; do Nascimento, E.M.; Rosado-de-Castro, P.H.; de Souza, S.A.L.; de SL Lima, R.; Pedrosa, R.C. Iodine-123 metaiodobenzylguanidine cardiac imaging as a method to detect early sympathetic neuronal dysfunction in chagasic patients with normal or borderline electrocardiogram and preserved ventricular function. *Clin. Nucl. Med.* **2011**, *36*, 757–761. [CrossRef]
37. Gadioli, L.P.; Miranda, C.H.; Pintya, A.O.; de Figueiredo, A.B.; Schmidt, A.; Maciel, B.C.; Marin-Neto, J.A.; Simoes, M.V. The severity of ventricular arrhythmia correlates with the extent of myocardial sympathetic denervation, but not with myocardial fibrosis extent in chronic Chagas cardiomyopathy: Chagas disease, denervation and arrhythmia. *J. Nucl. Cardiol.* **2018**, *25*, 75–83. [CrossRef]
38. James, O.G.; Christensen, J.D.; Wong, T.Z.; Borges-Neto, S.; Koweek, L.M. Utility of FDG PET/CT in inflammatory cardiovascular disease. *Radiographics* **2011**, *31*, 1271–1286. [CrossRef]
39. Blankstein, R.; Osborne, M.; Naya, M.; Waller, A.; Kim, C.K.; Murthy, V.L.; Kazemian, P.; Kwong, R.Y.; Tokuda, M.; Skali, H.; et al. Cardiac positron emission tomography enhances prognostic assessments of patients with suspected cardiac sarcoidosis. *J. Am. Coll. Cardiol.* **2014**, *63*, 329–336. [CrossRef]
40. Garg, G.; Cohen, S.; Neches, R.; Travin, M.I. Cardiac (18)F-FDG uptake in chagas disease. *J. Nucl. Cardiol.* **2016**, *23*, 321–325. [CrossRef]
41. Shapiro, H.; Meymandi, S.; Shivkumar, K.; Bradfield, J.S. Cardiac inflammation and ventricular tachycardia in Chagas disease. *HeartRhythm Case Rep.* **2017**, *3*, 392–395. [CrossRef] [PubMed]
42. Moll-Bernardes, R.J.; de Oliveira, R.S.; de Brito, A.S.X.; de Almeida, S.A.; Rosado-de-Castro, P.H.; de Sousa, A.S. Can PET/CT be useful in predicting ventricular arrhythmias in Chagas Disease? *J. Nucl. Cardiol.* **2020**, 1–4. [CrossRef] [PubMed]
43. Gormsen, L.C.; Haraldsen, A.; Kramer, S.; Dias, A.H.; Kim, W.Y.; Borghammer, P. A dual tracer (68)Ga-DOTANOC PET/CT and (18)F-FDG PET/CT pilot study for detection of cardiac sarcoidosis. *EJNMMI Res.* **2016**, *6*, 52. [CrossRef] [PubMed]

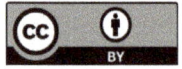

© 2020 by the authors. Licensee MDPI, Basel, Switzerland. This article is an open access article distributed under the terms and conditions of the Creative Commons Attribution (CC BY) license (http://creativecommons.org/licenses/by/4.0/).

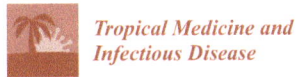

Opinion

Discussing the Score of Cardioembolic Ischemic Stroke in Chagas Disease

Fernanda de Souza Nogueira Sardinha Mendes *, Mauro Felippe Felix Mediano, Rudson Santos Silva, Sergio Salles Xavier, Pedro Emmanuel Alvarenga Americano do Brasil, Roberto Magalhães Saraiva, Alejandro Marcel Hasslocher-Moreno and Andrea Silvestre de Sousa

Instituto Nacional de Infectologia Evandro Chagas, Oswaldo Cruz Foundation (Fiocruz), Avenida Brasil 4365, Rio de Janeiro 21045-900, Brazil; mauro.mediano@ini.fiocruz.br (M.F.F.M.); rudson.santos@ini.fiocruz.br (R.S.S.); sergio.xavier@ini.fiocruz.br (S.S.X.); pedro.brasil@ini.fiocruz.br (P.E.A.A.d.B.); roberto.saraiva@ini.fiocruz.br (R.M.S.); alejandro.hasslocher@ini.fiocruz.br (A.M.H.-M.); andrea.silvestre@ini.fiocruz.br (A.S.d.S.)
* Correspondence: fernanda.sardinha@ini.fiocruz.br

Received: 28 February 2020; Accepted: 22 April 2020; Published: 26 May 2020

Abstract: Chagas disease is an important infection in Latin America but it is also reported in non-endemic countries all over the world. Around 30% of infected patients develop chronic Chagas cardiopathy, which is responsible for most poor outcomes, mainly heart failure, arrhythmias and thromboembolic events. Of all thromboembolic events, stroke is the most feared, due to the high probability of evolution to death or disability. Despite its importance, the actual incidence of cardioembolic ischemic stroke in Chagas disease is not completely known. The Instituto de Pesquisa Evandro Chagas/Fundação Oswaldo Cruz (IPEC-FIOCRUZ) score aims to propose prophylaxis strategies against cardioembolic ischemic stroke in Chagas disease based on clinical risk–benefit. To date, the IPEC-FIOCRUZ score is considered the best tool to identify patients for stroke prophylaxis in Chagas disease according the Latin American guideline and Brazilian consensus. It can prevent many cardioembolic strokes that would not be predicted, by applying the current recommendations to other cardiopathies. However, the IPEC-FIOCRUZ score still requires external validation to be used in different Chagas disease populations with an appropriate study design.

Keywords: Chagas disease; stroke; risk assessment

1. Chagas Disease and Stroke

Chagas disease (CD) is an important protozoan infection in Latin America where it remains one of the most important public health problems due to the high morbidity and mortality associated with the chronic cardiac form of the disease [1]. Nowadays, CD cases are also being reported worldwide due to international migration and autochthonous cases outside Latin America that may occur due to organ transplantation, blood transfusion and congenital transmission. The World Health Organization estimates that around six million people are infected by *Trypanosoma cruzi* [2]. Around 30% of infected patients develop the chronic cardiac form of the disease, responsible for most of the poor outcomes, mainly heart failure, arrhythmias and thromboembolic events [3,4]. Thromboembolic events in Chagas heart disease are more frequent than in other cardiopathies, even with similar degrees of systolic dysfunction [5], inferring that chagasic cardiopathy has a higher embolignic potential. For instance, a much higher frequency of chagasic stroke in patients without vascular risk factors is observed when compared to the non-Chagas cohort [6]. According to De Paiva Bezerra et al., in a 32-patient cohort, it was found that 87.5% had cardioembolic stroke, 9.4% had large intracranial artery atherosclerotic stroke and 3.1% had an undetermined cause [7]. Of all thromboembolic events, stroke is the most feared, due to the high probability of death or disability. Additionally, chagasic cardiopathy has unique characteristics such as apical aneurism, an important risk factor for cardioembolic events [6], which can limit the efficacy of prophylaxis in cardioembolic ischemic stroke (CIS). Thus, it is important to identify the main factors associated with an increased risk of cardioembolic ischemic stroke in CD and their mechanisms in order to propose tailored strategies to prevent it.

One study estimated that the annual incidence of CIS in a cohort of patients with CD was 3% in all subjects, and 4.4% in the high-risk subgroup, with a mean follow-up period of 5.5 years [8]. In a large Brazilian study [9], 24.4% of the stroke patients had positive serology for CD. A Colombian case-control study found similar results, detecting that *T. cruzi* infection was more frequent and statistically significant in stroke cases (24.4%) than controls (1.9%) [10]. Moreover, CD stroke patients had lower rates of cardiovascular risk factors but higher rates of multiple cerebrovascular events than non-Chagas patients did. In Colombia [11], CD was much more frequent among patients with stroke than in those with other diseases (OR = 12.13; 95% CI, 3.64 to 71.4). The cumulative incidence of death due to stroke among patients with CD was described to be 4.8% in a 10-year follow-up study [10], but new studies are needed to establish the mortality associated with stroke due to CD. Therefore, it is fundamental to identify strategies to prevent these events in patients with CD.

2. The IPEC-FIOCRUZ Stroke Score for Patients with Chagas Disease

The Instituto de Pesquisa Evandro Chagas/Fundação Oswaldo Cruz (IPEC-FIOCRUZ) score was developed, proposing prevention strategies for CIS in CD based on a risk–benefit analysis [9]. In the validation study, consecutive patients with positive serology for CD were followed for at least one year. The investigators studied two specific treatments: oral anticoagulation drugs and acetylsalicylic acid. The events were all cases of ischemic stroke or transient ischemic attack, defined as the cardioembolic type according to the Trial of Org 10172 in Acute Stroke Treatment (TOAST) classification [12]. Currently, the only group with a well-established proposal of prophylaxis, despite the CD diagnosis, is atrial fibrillation. The IPEC-FIOCRUZ score was built to fulfill the lack of knowledge of the individual risk–benefit of prophylaxis for cardioembolic stroke in the Chagas cardiopathy population not covered by the available scores. In this way, patients with previous ischemic stroke, intracavitary thrombus or atrial fibrillation were not included in this analysis because they already had a prophylaxis indication according to the in-force recommendations [13]. In this setting, fifty-two patients were observed, to evaluate the hemorrhagic risk of anticoagulation.

Four items were relevant in the IPEC-FIOCRUZ score: age >48 years, primary change of ventricular repolarization, systolic dysfunction and apical aneurysm of the left ventricle. The score ranges from zero to five points, and the group suggested primary prophylaxis with anticoagulants for those scoring ≥4 [6]. A total of 7.3% of the cohort was in a high-risk group (4–5 points) and 45% of them had the CIS diagnostic. This score was included in the Brazilian consensus and Latin American guideline for treatment of CD as an important strategy for detection of patients at increased risk of CIS [3,8,14].

Recently, Montanaro et al. [14] conducted a retrospective study that aimed to evaluate the performance of the IPEC-FIOCRUZ score in identifying patients at high risk of CIS. The authors included patients admitted to the SARAH Hospital of Rehabilitation from 2009 to 2013, diagnosed with ischemic stroke and CD. The mean time from ictus to inclusion was three years, and the mean follow-up time in the rehabilitation program was five years. By the TOAST etiological classification, 45% of the events were cardioembolic, 8.2% were atherothrombotic and in 45% the etiology of the event was not determined. The authors calculated the current IPEC-FIOCRUZ score of the patients and showed that 69.6% of the stroke patients had an IPEC-FIOCRUZ score of 1 or 2, and only 30.4% had a score of 3 or more. In addition, from those with cardioembolic etiology, 55% of patients were classified as low risk (IPEC-FIOCRUZ score <3). The authors concluded that more than half of the patients with cardioembolic strokes were misclassified as low risk and suggested that the current guidelines for stroke prevention in CD should be reviewed. However, there are several issues regarding population type, study design and data analysis that limited the authors' conclusions. The IPEC-FIOCRUZ score was built to predict individual cardioembolic risk and the benefit of each available treatment (i.e., warfarin and acetylsalicylic acid); however, Montanaro et al. [14] used this score in a population with known ischemic stroke from all etiologies (not only cardioembolic cases), in a retrospective analysis to check if the patients had a high score. As 55% of the cardioembolic events occurred in patients in the low-risk strata, Montanaro et al. supposed that if the score would have been applied before the occurrence of vascular ictus, the number of patients at risk would have been underestimated. However, the rationale used by the authors may be misleading, as discussed below. There were also no data regarding the previous use of anticoagulant or antiplatelet therapy by the patients who suffered stroke.

The purpose of a risk assessment tool (i.e., risk score) is to assess individual risk and propose recommendations of actions according to the estimated risk. In most cases, the group with the highest individual risk is much smaller than the low-risk group, which results in a higher absolute number of outcomes in the low-risk group. This apparent paradox has been described for many years in relation to sudden death [15,16]. Although the patients at high relative risk for sudden cardiac death can be identified by their risk factors, the greatest number of sudden death cases occurs in patients not previously determined to be at high risk. This paradox makes it difficult to adopt preventive measures on a large scale [17]. Using the example of Geoffrey Rose in his paper [18], when we think of the occurrence of Down's syndrome births in regards to maternal age, younger mothers are at minimal risk; but because they are the majority, they generate half the cases. The lesson is that "a large number of people with small risk may give rise to more cases of disease than the small number who are at high risk". If we think with this approach in cardioembolic stroke in CD, most of the cases are in the low-risk population. This is one of the reasons why it is not right to validate the risk score by applying it to the prevalent cases. To validate a score, we need to apply it to the whole population that is at risk of the event—in this case, people with CD free of cardioembolic stroke—and compare the predicted events with the observed ones. This will enable the estimation of discrimination and calibration measures.

The second important issue: Is it appropriate to include all patients with cardioembolic stroke, even those with previous stroke and atrial fibrillation, and apply the IPEC-FIOCRUZ score? These predictors were not included in the score because they already had an indication for stroke prophylaxis before the risk assessment. From a practical point of view, it does not make sense to use a score in helping to decide whether to prescribe anticoagulants when the patient should already be taking this therapy [19].

3. Perspectives for Scoring Stroke Risk in Chagas Disease

The IPEC-FIOCRUZ score was validated in a single center with a relatively small sample size. Therefore, it requires external validation to be used in different populations with CD, but an appropriate study design is necessary. The area under the Receiver Operating Characteristic (ROC) curve of this model was 0.90 (95% CI 0.86 to 0.94), which is the best parameter to evaluate score accuracy until an external validation in a different cohort is done. There are increasingly acceptable standards in the literature regarding development, validation and update of prediction/decision models [20]. A study to validate the IPEC-FIOCRUZ stroke score should include subjects with CD, initially stroke-free, but at potential risk of stroke occurrence in the future. Additionally, the subjects should represent the population where a decision to introduce preventive therapy is required. A prediction score in this case should be applied when observation starts, where potential courses of actions are in discussion, and not for those that should be already taking prophylactic therapy, i.e., for previous cardioembolic stroke, intracavitary thrombus or atrial fibrillation. Later, the discrimination ability and calibration would be estimated when comparing the predictions with the observed events.

The validation and update of useful prediction/decision models are always advisable, mainly where the model may be applicable in several different settings (e.g., rural cohorts, non-endemic countries, different health units, etc.). However, this effort should follow standards currently acceptable for an appropriate interpretation. These appropriate validation studies are welcome and expected for all models of a devastating neglected disease.

4. Conclusions

Until now, the IPEC-FIOCRUZ score remains the best stroke prophylaxis tool in CD according to the Latin American guideline and Brazilian consensus [3,8], which is capable of identifying patients at risk and avoiding cardioembolic strokes that would not be avoided by applying the usual recommendations for stroke prophylaxis in other cardiopathies.

Author Contributions: All authors contributed to the preparation of this opinion. All authors have read and agreed to the published version of the manuscript.

Funding: This research received no external funding.

Acknowledgments: The authors thank the clinical and administrative staff from Evandro Chagas National Institute of Infectious Disease for their support.

Conflicts of Interest: The authors declare no conflict of interest.

References

1. Pérez-Molina, J.A.; Molina, I. Chagas disease. *Lancet* **2018**, *391*, 82–94. [CrossRef]
2. Chagas disease in Latin America: An epidemiological update based on 2010 estimates. *Wkly. Epidemiol. Rec.* **2015**, *90*, 33–43.
3. Andrade, J.P.; Marin Neto, J.A.; Paola, A.A.V.; Vilas-Boas, F.; Oliveira, G.M.M.; Bacal, F.; Bocchi, E.A.; Almeida, D.R.; Filho, A.A.F.; Da Consolação Vieira Moreira, M.; et al. I Latin American Guidelines for the diagnosis and treatment of Chagas' heart disease: Executive summary. *Arq. Bras. Cardiol.* **2011**, *96*, 434–442. [CrossRef]
4. Ribeiro, A.L.; Nunes, M.P.; Teixeira, M.M.; Rocha, M.O.C. Diagnosis and management of Chagas disease and cardiomyopathy. *Nat. Rev. Cardiol.* **2012**, *9*, 576–589. [CrossRef] [PubMed]
5. Dries, D.L.; Rosenberg, Y.D.; Waclawiw, M.A.; Domanski, M.J. Ejection fraction and risk of thromboembolic events in patients with systolic dysfunction and sinus rhythm: Evidence for gender differences in the studies of left ventricular dysfunction trials. *J. Am. Coll. Cardiol.* **1997**, *29*, 1074–1080. [CrossRef]
6. Da Matta, J.A.; Aras, R., Jr.; De Macedo, C.R.B.; Da Cruz, C.G.; Netto, E.M. Stroke correlates in chagasic and non-chagasic cardiomyopathies. *PLoS ONE* **2012**, *7*, e35116. [CrossRef] [PubMed]
7. De Paiva Bezerra, R.; De Miranda Alves, M.A.; Conforto, A.B.; Rodrigues, D.L.G.; Silva, G.S. Etiological Classification of Stroke in Patients with Chagas Disease Using TOAST, Causative Classification System TOAST, and ASCOD Phenotyping. *J. Stroke Cerebrovasc. Dis.* **2017**, *26*, 2864–2869. [CrossRef]
8. Dias, J.C.; Ramos, A.N.; Gontijo, E.D.; Luquetti, A.; Shikanai-Yasuda, M.A.; Coura, J.R.; Torres, R.M.; Melo, J.R.C.; Almeida, E.A.; Oliveira, W.; et al. 2nd Brazilian Consensus on Chagas Disease, 2015. *Rev. Soc. Bras. Med. Trop.* **2016**, *49* (Suppl. 1), 3–60. [CrossRef]
9. Sousa, A.S.; Xavier, S.S.; De Freitas, G.R.; Hasslocher-Moreno, A.M. Prevention strategies of cardioembolic ischemic stroke in Chagas' disease. *Arq. Bras. Cardiol.* **2008**, *91*, 306–310. [CrossRef] [PubMed]
10. Leon-Sarmiento, F.E.; Mendoza, E.; Torres-Hillera, M.; Pinto, N.; Prada, J.; Silva, C.A.; Vera, S.J.; Castillo, E.; Valderrama, V.; Prada, D.; et al. Trypanosoma cruzi-associated cerebrovascular disease: A case-control study in Eastern Colombia. *J. Neurol. Sci.* **2004**, *217*, 61–64. [CrossRef] [PubMed]
11. Carod-Artal, F.J.; Vargas, A.P.; Melo, M.; Horan, T.A. American trypanosomiasis (Chagas' disease): An unrecognised cause of stroke. *J. Neurol. Neurosurg. Psychiatry* **2003**, *74*, 516–518. [CrossRef] [PubMed]
12. Ay, H.; Furie, K.L.; Singhal, A.; Smith, W.S.; Sorensen, A.G.; Koroshetz, W.J. An evidence-based causative classification system for acute ischemic stroke. *Ann. Neurol.* **2005**, *58*, 688–697. [CrossRef] [PubMed]
13. Fuster, V.; Rydén, L.E.; Cannom, D.S.; Crijns, H.J.; Curtis, A.B.; Ellenbogen, K.A.; Halperin, J.L.; Le Heuzey, J.-Y.; Kay, G.N.; Lowe, J.E.; et al. ACC/AHA/ESC 2006 Guidelines for the Management of Patients with Atrial Fibrillation: A report of the American College of Cardiology/American Heart Association Task Force on Practice Guidelines and the European Society of Cardiology Committee for Practice Guidelines (Writing Committee to Revise the 2001 Guidelines for the Management of Patients With Atrial Fibrillation): Developed in collaboration with the European Heart Rhythm Association and the Heart Rhythm Society. *Circulation* **2006**, *114*, e257–e354. [PubMed]

14. Montanaro, V.V.; Da Silva, C.M.; De Viana Santos, C.V.; Lima, I.M.I.R.; Negrão, E.M.; De Freitas, G.R. Ischemic stroke classification and risk of embolism in patients with Chagas disease. *J. Neurol.* **2016**, *263*, 2411–2415. [CrossRef] [PubMed]
15. Podrid, P.J.; Myerburg, R.J. Epidemiology and stratification of risk for sudden cardiac death. *Clin. Cardiol.* **2005**, *28*, I3–I11. [CrossRef] [PubMed]
16. Myerburg, R.J.; Spooner, P.M. Opportunities for sudden death prevention: Directions for new clinical and basic research. *Cardiovasc. Res.* **2001**, *50*, 177–185. [CrossRef]
17. Rassi, A.; Rassi, S.G. Sudden death in Chagas' disease. *Arq. Bras. Cardiol.* **2001**, *76*, 75–96. [CrossRef] [PubMed]
18. Rose, G. Sick individuals and sick populations. *Int. J. Epidemiol.* **2001**, *30*, 427–432. [CrossRef] [PubMed]
19. Johnston, S.C.; Rothwell, P.M.; Nguyen-Huynh, M.N.; Giles, M.F.; Elkins, J.S.; Bernstein, A.L.; Sidney, S. Validation and refinement of scores to predict very early stroke risk after transient ischaemic attack. *Lancet* **2007**, *369*, 283–292. [CrossRef]
20. Moons, K.G.; De Groot, J.A.; Bouwmeester, W.; Vergouwe, Y.; Mallett, S.; Altman, D.G.; Reitsma, J.B.; Collins, G.S. Critical appraisal and data extraction for systematic reviews of prediction modelling studies: The CHARMS checklist. *PLoS Med.* **2014**, *11*, e1001744. [CrossRef] [PubMed]

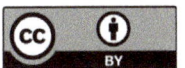

© 2020 by the authors. Licensee MDPI, Basel, Switzerland. This article is an open access article distributed under the terms and conditions of the Creative Commons Attribution (CC BY) license (http://creativecommons.org/licenses/by/4.0/).

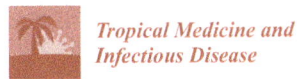

Case Report

Effects of Meglumine Antimoniate Treatment on Cytokine Production in a Patient with Mucosal Leishmaniasis and Chagas Diseases Co-Infection

Karine Rezende-Oliveira [1,†], Cesar Gómez-Hernández [2,†,*], Marcos Vinícius da Silva [3], Rafael Faria de Oliveira [4], Juliana Reis Machado [5], Luciana de Almeida Silva Teixeira [6], Lúcio Roberto Cançado Castellano [7], Dalmo Correia [6] and Virmondes Rodrigues [2]

1. Laboratory of Biomedical Sciences, Federal University of Uberlândia, Ituiutaba, Minas Gerais CEP 38304-402, Brazil; karinerezende@ufu.br
2. Laboratory of Immunology, Federal University of Triângulo Mineiro, Uberaba, Minas Gerais CEP 38025-180, Brazil; virmondes.junior@uftm.edu.br
3. Laboratory of Parasitology, Federal University of Triângulo Mineiro, Uberaba, Minas Gerais CEP 38025-180, Brazil; marcos.silva@uftm.edu.br
4. Laboratory of Clinical Analysis, Professional Education Center, Federal University of Triângulo Mineiro, Uberaba, Minas Gerais CEP 38025-404, Brazil; rafael.oliveira@uftm.edu.br
5. Discipline of General Pathology, Federal University of Triângulo Mineiro, Uberaba, Minas Gerais CEP 38025-200, Brazil; juliana.machado@uftm.edu.br
6. Infectious Diseases Division, Federal University of Triângulo Mineiro, Uberaba, Minas Gerais CEP 38025-180, Brazil; lalmeidas@terra.com.br (L.d.A.S.T.); dalmo@mednet.com.br (D.C.)
7. Human Immunology Research and Education Group, Technical School of Health of Federal University of Paraíba, João Pessoa, Paraíba CEP 58059-900, Brazil; luciocastellano@gmail.com
* Correspondence: cesar_cgh@hotmail.com
† These authors contributed equally to this work.

Received: 10 March 2020; Accepted: 14 April 2020; Published: 2 May 2020

Abstract: The influence of antimoniate treatment on specific anti-protozoan T-cell responses was evaluated in a 48-year-old male patient diagnosed with mucosal leishmaniasis and Chagas disease infection. Before and after treatment, PBMC (peripheral blood mononuclear cells) were cultured in the absence or presence of *Leishmania braziliensis* or *Trypanosoma cruzi* live parasites, their soluble antigens, or PHA (phytohaemagglutinin). Cytokines were measured and Treg (T regulatory) cell percentages were quantified. Before treatment, PBMC were able to produce higher amounts of TNF-α, IL-6 (Interleukin-6), and IL-10 (Interleukin-10) but lower amounts of IL-12 (Interleukin-12) in response to culture stimulation. However, after treatment, there was a down-modulation of TNF-α, IL-6, and IL-10 cytokines but an up-modulation in IL-12 production. PBMC had the ability to produce TNF-α only against live parasites or PHA. There was an overall decrease of circulating Treg cells after treatment. In mixed Leishmaniasis and Chagas disease infection, treatment with antimoniate could modulate immune responses toward a more protective profile to both diseases.

Keywords: mucosal leishmaniasis; Chagas disease; co-infection; antimoniate therapy

1. Introduction

American Tegumentary Leishmaniasis (ATL) and Chagas disease (CD) are protozoan infections caused by *Leishmania sp.* and *Trypanosoma cruzi*, respectively. These neglected diseases occur in the tropics with an overlapping distribution of endemic areas, especially in South America [1]. Both diseases show diverse clinical presentations varying from localized cutaneous form to mucosal manifestations (ML) for ATL and from asymptomatic individuals to patients with digestive abnormalities to patients with severe heart failure for CD [1]. Immune response against CD is characterized by pro-inflammatory cytokine production, while in ATL, significant anti-inflammatory cytokine production has been observed. Furthermore, a particular role developed by T regulatory cells (Tregs) has been considered. Treatments for both diseases are very complex and some effects of the first-choice drugs remain unclear. Drugs indicated for CD treatment are nifurtimox and benznidazole, both presenting an average cure rate from 80% in acute disease to less than 20% in chronic infections [2]. In the case of ML, the pentavalent antimonial drugs still are the first option, although they present important side effects and variable efficacy. Amphotericin B and pentamidine are also suggested; however, their cost and the toxicity observed in clinical studies restrict their use in ATL treatment [3].

There are few reports in the literature providing evidences of patients with suspected or confirmed mixed infections [4–9]. Usually, these reports explore the cross-reactivity among parasite's antigens used in serodiagnostic by ELISA (Enzyme-Linked Immunosorbent Assay) kits or the establishment of a more specific molecular tool rather than patients' clinical status. However, the immunological responses of patients with mixed *L. braziliensis* and *T. cruzi* infections still need to be evaluated. In this context, we aimed to evaluate the influence of treatment with meglumine antimoniate on the specific anti-protozoan T-cell response in a case of mixed mucosal leishmaniasis and Chagas disease infection.

2. Case Report

A 48-year-old male was admitted to the Clinical Hospital of Federal University of Triângulo Mineiro, with a four-month progressive mucosal lesion on his septum. The patient reported itching and occasional epistaxis. At the time of admission, physical examination revealed a septal perforation and a roundish scar on his left leg as a consequence of a previous ulcerative lesion spontaneously healed 3 years ago. Immunohistochemical analysis of the nasal biopsy was positive for *Leishmania* amastigotes, whereas histology was negative for *Mycobacterium sp.* and fungi (Figure 1A). The patient presented normal blood pressure and heart rate. Chest and abdominal radiography (Figure 1C) as well as abdominal ultrasound were normal. Electrocardiography (ECG) revealed a T-wave inversion on V4, V5, V6, and diffuse ventricular repolarization abnormalities (Figure 1B). Transesophageal echocardiography demonstrated a left ventricular ejection fraction (EF) = 50% and shortening fraction of 26%, right and left atrial and right ventricular normal dimensions. Increased left ventricular size with decreased systolic performance and diffuse hypokinesis. As a result of the patient's origin from an endemic area for Chagas disease and due to his altered ECG, serology for *T. cruzi* was performed and was positive in all tests: indirect hemagglutination assay, indirect immunofluorescence, and TESA-blot (BioMérieux, Brazil) is an immunoblotting assay that uses secreted and excreted trypomastigote antigens (Figure 1E). In order to discriminate from a serological cross-reactivity with *Leishmania* antigens, the molecular detection of *T. cruzi* DNA was performed by PCR (Figure 1D) using the following primers that amplify a 330 bp fragment: 121 (5′-AAA TAA TGT ACG GGK GAG ATG CAT GA-3′) and 122 (5′-GGT TCG ATT GGG GTT GGT GTA ATA TA-3′) [10]. Serology for HIV was negative. The patient was diagnosed with mucosal leishmaniasis (ML) and Chagas disease co-infection, chronic fase with cardiac form (functional class II of the New York Heart Association). The patient's treatment was in accordance with standard Brazilian Ministry of Health clinical practice. Meglumine antimoniate (Glucantime®) treatment was started for 30 days, being 20 mg Sb + 5/kg/day for 13 days and 15 mg Sb + 5/kg/day for 17 days due to detectable hepatotoxicity. The patient remained hospitalized for 40 days and was discharged and sent to the Plastic Surgery Division for evaluation and outpatient follow up.

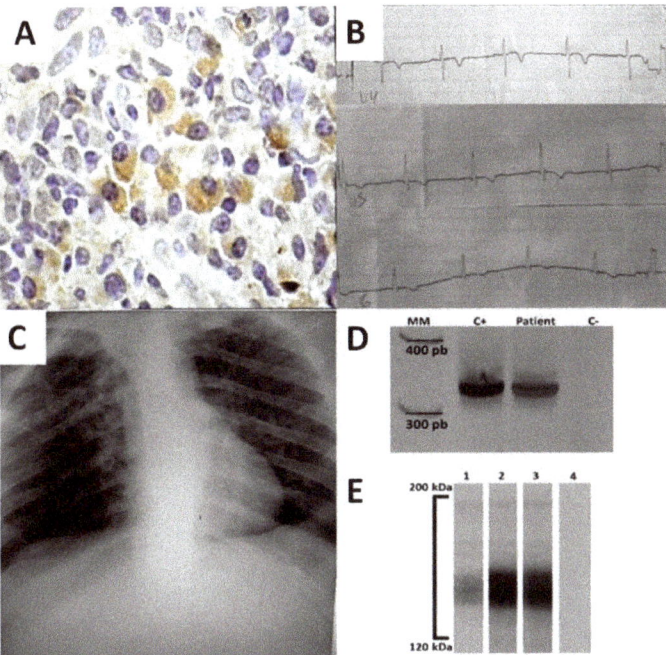

Figure 1. Clinical data and laboratorial findings of a patient with Chagas disease and Leishmaniasis co-infection. (**A**) Immunohistochemistry for the detection of Leishmania's antigens in nasal septum biopsy. Brown areas indicate the presence of *Leishmania sp.* antigens (**B**) Electrocardiographic alterations showing V4, V5, and V6 derivations with T-wave inversion indicating chronic chagasic cardiopathy. (**C**) Chest radiography. (**D**) Molecular detection of *T. cruzi* DNA using specific primers 121–122 by PCR. Lines MM- 100 bp molecular marker; C+ positive control; patient-patient's sample; C− negative control. (**E**) TESA-blot positive for *T. cruzi* before and after treatment of patient. Lines 1—positive control; 2—patient's sample before treatment; 3—patient's sample after treatment; 4—negative control.

Venous blood was collected in two different time periods: (1) at the moment of patient's admission, just after clinical evaluation and before any treatment regimen and (2) at the end of specific treatment for mucocutaneous leishmaniasis (40-day period of Glucantime® regimen). In both periods, peripheral blood mononuclear cells (PBMC) were separated using Ficoll-Paque™ Plus gradient (GE Health Care, Uppsala, Sweden) and cultured in RPMI 1640 (GIBCO, Grand Island, NY, USA) in 8 different culture conditions: medium alone, 2 ug/mL Phytohaemagglutinin (Sigma, St. Louis, MO, USA), 3:1 *T cruzi* (Y strain) or 3:1 *L. braziliensis* (Lb2904 strain) live parasites, as well as 5 ug/mL *T. cruzi* and 5 ug/mL *L. braziliensis* soluble proteins, in a 5% CO_2 atmosphere at 37 °C for 24 h, as described elsewhere [11,12]. The supernatants were used for cytokine quantification, IL-6, IL-10, TNF-α and IL-12, by ELISA assay as previously described [11,13]. Briefly, for each cytokine quantification, 96-well flat-bottomed polystyrene microtiter ELISA plates (Costar, Corning, NY) were coated with indicated monoclonal antibody 1 µg/mL (BD Pharmingen, San Diego, CA, USA). Non-reactive sites in the wells were blocked with 2% BSA (bovine serum albumin) in coating buffer. Culture supernatants were added at 100 µL/well and incubated for 2 h at room temperature. Horseradish peroxidase conjugated anti-cytokine monoclonal antibodies (BD Pharmingen, San Diego, CA, USA) were added at 1 µg/mL. After, TMB (tetramethylbenzidine) substrate solution (BD Pharmingen, San Diego, CA, USA) was used for assay revelation, which was read on a microplate reader at 750 nm (Bio-Rad Microplate reader-Benchmark, Hercules, CA, USA), and sample concentrations were determined by simple regression over a standard curve and values were obtained in pg/mL (Figure 2A–D). The results expressed on Figure 2E,H were elaborated considering the equation:

$$\frac{(\text{cytokine levels in stimulated cells} - \text{cytokine levels in medium alone})}{\text{cytokine levels in medium alone}}$$

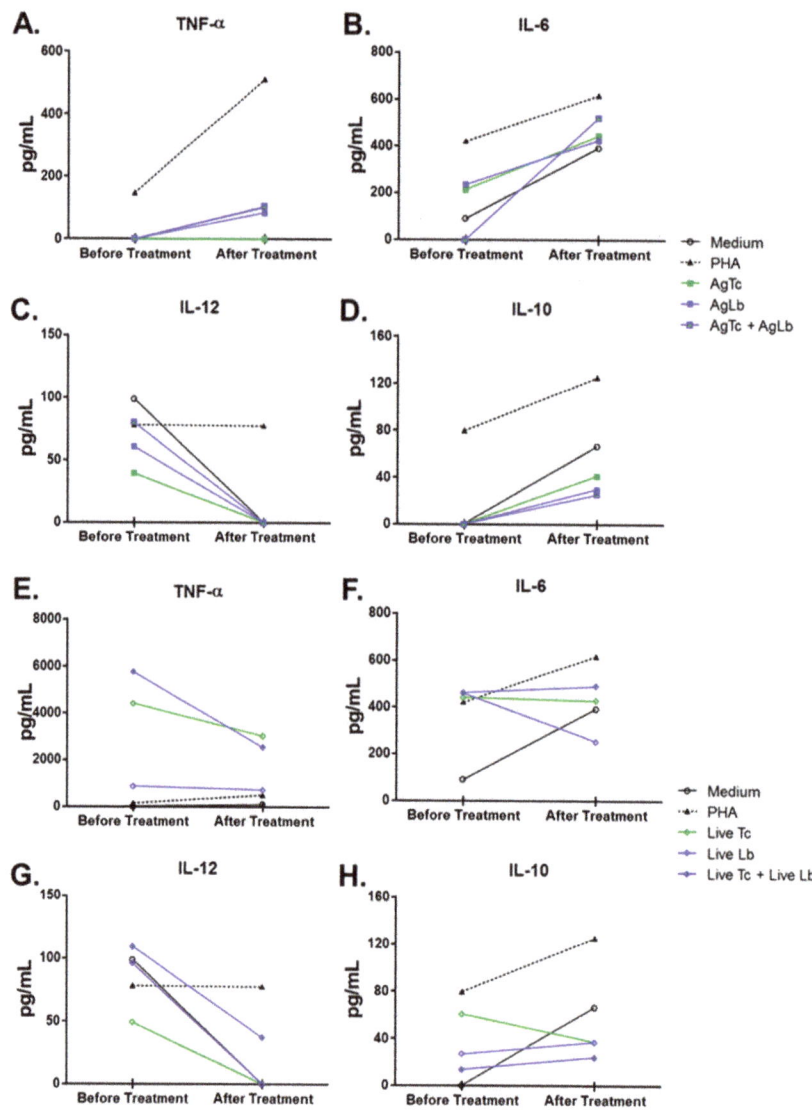

Figure 2. Cytokine's production by peripheral blood mononuclear cells (PBMC) stimulated in vitro before and after patient's treatment with meglumine antimoniate. Graph (**A–D**) depicts the level of (**A**) TNF-α; (**B**) IL-6; (**C**) IL-10, and (**D**) IL-12 detected by ELISA in culture supernatants before and after treatment. Graphs (**E–H**) depict the fold induction capacity of antigens and live parasites on cytokine production over basal stimulation (medium alone). Open bars represent results before treatment and full bars represent results after treatment.

Another fraction of isolated PBMC was subjected to ex vivo immunophenotyping. Cells were suspended in 100 µL of Hanks' balanced salt solution (Sigma, St. Louis, MO, USA) at a final concentration of 5×10^5 cells/mL and incubated with 5 µL of fluorochrome-conjugated antibodies (BD Pharmingen, San Diego, CA, USA) against the following surface markers: CD4-PE-Cy7 (clone RPA-T4) and CD25-FITC (clone PC61). For intracellular staining, cells were permeabilized with BD Cytofix/Cytoperm™ Plus (BD Biosciences) and then incubated with 10 µl of the FoxP3-PE (clone 259D/C7) antibody. Multiparameter flow cytometry was performed using a FACScalibur flow cytometer (Becton Dickinson, Mountain View, CA, USA) compensated with single fluorochromes. Data were analyzed using Cell Quest Pro software (Becton Dickinson). Dead cells were omitted by side scatter/forward scatter (SSC/FSC) gating, and isotype-matched control antibodies were used to determine background levels of staining (Figure 3).

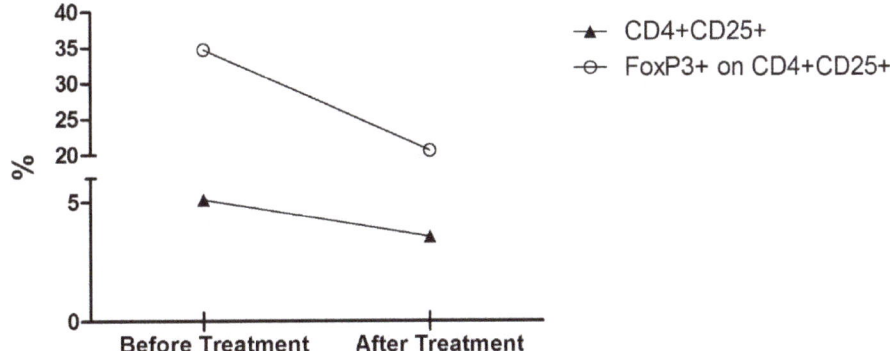

Figure 3. Percentage of circulating cells with T regulatory phenotype before and after treatment. Graph depicts the ex vivo percentage of CD4$^+$CD25$^+$ T cells (▲) and the percentage of Foxp3$^+$ cells on CD4$^+$CD25$^+$ T cells subpopulation (○) from the patient's PBMC collected before and after treatment with meglumine antimoniate.

3. Results and Discussion

The occurrence of an overlapping distribution of ATL and CD in endemic areas would be detrimental for a large number of patients to be diagnosed with mixed infections [1]. However, few reports on the literature demonstrated these two diseases affecting the same group of patients at the same time [4–9]. All these studies were drowning to promote accurate diagnostic tests that are capable of eliminating serological cross-reactivity between *Leishmania sp.* and *T. cruzi*. Despite their relevancy to the field, some important issues still need attention. The present study aimed to deal with one of the missing aspects by evaluating the potential effects of meglumine antimoniate treatment on cellular immune responses of a patient with ATL/CD co-infection. Soon after the case definition but still before any treatment, it was decided to analyze the patient's immunological response by evaluating the production of some cytokines (TNF-α, IL-6, IL-10, and IL-12) that might have an impact in both ML and CD pathogenesis. The blood sample was collected before the patient's treatment with meglumine antimoniate and just before patient discharge; another venous blood sample was collected and processed in order to evaluate the possible immunomodulatory effects of treatment.

The capacity of cells to respond to the various stimuli was affected by the treatment with meglumine antimoniate; there seemed to be TNF-α increasing levels when cells were stimulated with AgLb and AgLb + Lc and decreasing production with stimuli of live Lc and live Lc + Lb. In contrast, stimulation with live parasites induced high levels of TNF-α and antigens (Figure 2A). IL6 increased in production when stimulated with parasite antigens and decreased when stimulated with live Lb (Figure 2B). There were decreasing levels of IL-12 with any stimuli (Figure 2C). The IL10 had increased production except with live Tc stimuli. Considering the importance of circulating Treg cells in patients with one of each disease when presented alone [13–15], it was decided to evaluate the effect of the meglumine antimoniate treatment over Treg cell counts in this patient, presenting a mixed infection. There was an overall decrease in the number of $CD4^+CD25^{High+}$ T cells as well as in the percentage of $Foxp3^+$ cells within this population after treatment.

In general, treatment with meglumine antimoniate seemed not to induce changes in TNF-α levels, thus increasing the production of IL-6 and IL-10 and decreasing the levels of IL-12 (Figure 2A–D). The capacity of cells to respond to the various stimuli was also observed when the basal levels were subtracted, considering the cultured cells in medium alone (Figure 2E,H). Before treatment, patient's peripheral blood cells were stimulated by live parasites, and their soluble proteins or PHA produced higher levels of TNF-α, IL-6, and IL-10 but lower IL-12 cytokines in comparison to culture medium alone (basal production). However, after treatment, there was a remarkable change in the ability of cells to respond to stimuli; this was observed by the down-modulation of TNF-α, IL-6, and IL-10 cytokines but the up-modulation in IL-12 production, which recovered the ability to achieve baseline levels. Cytokine levels were quite often detected at equal or below the amount measured in a medium condition alone. Interestingly, cultured cells still had the ability to produce TNF-α only against live parasites (Live-Tc and Live-Lb) or phytohaemagglutinin (PHA), but not against parasite antigens (Figure 2E). Considering the importance of circulating Treg cells in patients with one of each disease when presented alone [13–15], it was decided to evaluate the effect of the meglumine antimoniate treatment over Treg cell counts in this patient, presenting a mixed infection. There was an overall decrease in the number of $CD4^+CD25^{High+}$ T cells as well as in the percentage of $Foxp3^+$ cells within this population after treatment.

There is strong evidence showing that an unbalanced production of inflammatory/modulatory cytokines is crucial to tissue damage and worse prognosis in both ML and CD. Studies conducted in ATL patients with localized cutaneous lesions (LCL) had shown that treatment with meglumine antimoniate decreased the IL-4 and IL-10 production by antigen-stimulated PBMC [11,13,16,17]. The reactive $CD4^+$ T cells still produced significant IL-10 levels, even after the treatment of ATL patients [17]. In addition, it has been shown that genetic polymorphisms in the promoter region of the *il10* gene induced elevated amounts of IL-10 independently of IFN-γ (Interferon-γ) production in patients with LCL [13]. Increased IFN-γ and TNF-α production was observed in both $CD4^+$ and $CD8^+$ T cells post-chemotherapy [17]. Higher levels of specific anti-*Leishmania* $CD4^+$ and $CD8^+$ T cells had been observed in patients with ML in comparison to individuals with LCL. The IFN-γ production did not change in ML after treatment and was always higher than that observed in patients with CL [16]. Again, a functional polymorphism in the IFN-γ gene induced lower INF-γ production in ATL patients. However, the allele frequencies studied could not distinguish between healthy control subjects and ATL patients or between CL and ML forms of the disease, nor could it be associated to disease susceptibility or worse prognosis [18]. On the other hand, polymorphism in the intron region of the TNF gene was associated to elevated cytokine levels in sera from ATL patients in comparison to healthy subjects. In addition, it was associated with a higher risk for mucosal involvement in infected patients [19]. These data indicate that strong TNF-α response in treated patients might predict unfavorable outcomes in the evolution from CL to ML forms of the disease, whereas a down-modulation in IL-4 and IL-10 production would play an important role in infection control and disease better prognosis. Our results reinforces data regarding the role of meglumine antimoniate treatment decreasing TNF-α and IL-10 production in the ML/CD patient, which would be beneficial to clinical cure and disease remission. Considering the Treg cells, it has been demonstrated that this population recovered from the infected skin of LCL patients produces IL-10 and exerts an immunomodulatory phenotype that is capable of inhibiting the proliferation of CD4+ effector T cells [14]. Patients with active LCL lesions presented a higher percentage of circulating $CD4^+CD25^+Foxp3^+$ T cells in comparison to both patients with healed lesions and endemic area inhabitants with a resistant phenotype [13]. The decrease in the percentage of circulating $CD4^+CD25^+Foxp3^+$ T cells observed in the case related here indicates that successful healing would be partially dependent on the decrease of this cell population induced by the meglumine antimoniate chemotherapy. Previous work has shown that treatment with meglumine antimoniate interferes with phagocytosis in monocytes from LCL patients [20]. The authors reported that meglumine antimoniate increased IFN-γ serum levels, while it up-regulated the phagocytic function of monocytes in association with the increase in production of TNF-α but not IL-10 by these cells. Together with our results, it suggests a strong immunomodulatory effect of meglumine antimoniate in distinct cell subsets.

Chagasic patients with an indeterminate form or presenting less aggressive cardiomyopathy have an increase in IL-10 and IL-17 production as well as in the number and in the suppressive function of $CD4^+CD25^{high}Foxp3^+$ Treg cells than patients with severe cardiomyopathy. Moreover, it was shown that Treg cells from cardiac patients were able to produce elevated levels of IL-6, IFN-γ, and TNF-α and are unable to modulate the TNF-α and IFN-γ production from leukocytes [15,21]. Interestingly, it has been observed that the proper TNF-α itself induces IL-10 production in human monocytes as a negative feedback loop [22]. Higher cytokine production together with genetic polymorphisms in the promoter region of the TNF-α gene was associated with human infection with *T. cruzi* [23]. An in situ analysis of cytokine production in the heart tissues of subjects who had died during the chronic phase of Chagas disease suggested a pivotal role of TNF-α and IFN-γ-producing cells in promoting heart failure and fibrosis [24,25]. One might infer that circulating Treg cells would bring protection to indeterminate patients. Thus, the fact that these cells are not enough to dampen the inflammatory response in more severe cardiac forms of the disease suggests that diminishing the levels of Treg cells in cardiac patients would not be immediately associated with a worse prognosis. In this way, our results seem to be promising by the fact that treatment decreased the percentage of circulating $CD4^+CD25^+Foxp3^+$ T cells, concomitantly to the decreased ability of leukocytes to produce TNF-α, IL-6, and IL-10 in response to live parasites or their antigens. Live trypomastigotes of the same *T. cruzi* Y strain used in our study were able to induce TNF-α and IL-12 but not IL-10 production in PBMC of CD seronegative healthy individuals [12]. This suggests an important *in vivo* clonal expansion of parasite-specific IL-10-producing T cells.

The administration of antimoniate may induce cardiac alterations that are observed in ECG [26]. This would be detrimental to patients already presenting altered ECG. However, in the patient studied here, who was diagnosed with Chagas disease, the treatment with meglumine antimoniate did not promote any enhancement on cardiac commitment already existent. Additional studies with a larger number of patients are needed to evaluate a possible role of meglumine antimoniate in chagasic cardiomyopathy.

4. Conclusions

The results presented here highlight the importance of a complete clinical and laboratory investigation of patients coming from geographical regions that present overlapping endemic areas for parasitic diseases. In case of a mixed Leishmaniasis and Chagas disease infection, treatment with meglumine antimoniate would be beneficial to modulate patient's immune responses toward a more protective profile to both diseases.

Author Contributions: Conceptualization, K.R.-O., C.G.-H., L.d.A.S.T. and V.R.; methodology, K.R.-O, C.G.-H., M.V.D.S., R.F.d.O., V.R.; software, K.R.-O., C.G.-H. and M.V.D.S.; validation, K.R.-O., C.G.-H., M.V.D.S., R.F.d.O., J.R.M. and V.R.; formal analysis, K.R.-O., C.G.-H., M.V.D.S., R.F.d.O., J.R.M., L.R.C.C. and V.R.; investigation, K.R.-O., C.G.-H., M.V.D.S., L.d.A.S.T., L.R.C.C., D.C. and V.R.; resources, K.R.-O. and C.G.-H.; data curation, K.R.-O, C.G.-H. and M.V.D.S.; writing—original draft preparation, K.R.O, C.G.-H., M.V.D.S., L.d.A.S.T., L.R.C.C., D.C. and V.C.; writing—review and editing, K.R.-O., C.G.-H. and V.R.; visualization, K.R.-O., C.G.-H., M.V.D.S. and V.R.; supervision, K.R.-O., C.G.-H. and V.R.; project administration, K.R.-O., C.G.-H., V.R.; funding acquisition, V.R. All authors have read and agreed to the published version of the manuscript.

Funding: This research received no external funding.

Acknowledgments: Authors are in debt to all technical staff of the division of immunology and infectious diseases at the Federal University of Triângulo Mineiro.

Conflicts of Interest: The authors declare that they have no conflicts of interest.

References

1. WHO. *Sustaining the Drive to Overcome the Global Impact of Neglected Tropical Diseases: Second WHO Report on Neglected Diseases*; WHO: Geneva, Switzerland, 2013; p. 138.
2. Coura, J.R.; Borges-Pereira, J. Chagas disease. What is known and what should be improved: A systemic review. *Rev. Soc. Bras. Med. Trop.* **2012**, *45*, 286–296. [CrossRef] [PubMed]
3. Reithinger, R.; Dujardin, J.C.; Louzir, H.; Pirmez, C.; Alexander, B.; Brooker, S. Cutaneous leishmaniasis. *Lancet Infect. Dis.* **2007**, *7*, 581–596. [CrossRef]
4. Malchiodi, E.L.; Chiaramonte, M.G.; Taranto, N.J.; Zwirner, N.W.; Margni, R.A. Cross-reactivity studies and differential serodiagnosis of human infections caused by Trypanosoma cruzi and Leishmania spp; use of immunoblotting and ELISA with a purified antigen (Ag163B6). *Clin. Exp. Immunol.* **1994**, *97*, 417–423. [CrossRef] [PubMed]
5. Chiaramonte, M.G.; Zwirner, N.W.; Caropresi, S.L.; Taranto, N.J.; Malchiodi, E.L. Trypanosoma cruzi and Leishmania spp. human mixed infection. *Am. J. Trop. Med. Hyg.* **1996**, *54*, 271–273. [CrossRef] [PubMed]
6. Chiaramonte, M.G.; Frank, F.M.; Furer, G.M.; Taranto, N.J.; Margni, R.A.; Malchiodi, E.L. Polymerase chain reaction reveals Trypanosoma cruzi infection suspected by serology in cutaneous and mucocutaneous leishmaniasis patients. *Acta Trop.* **1999**, *72*, 295–308. [CrossRef]
7. Passos, V.M.; Volpini, A.C.; Braga, E.M.; Lacerda, P.A.; Ouaissi, A.; Lima-Martins, M.V.; Krettli, A.U. Differential serodiagnosis of human infections caused by Trypanosoma cruzi and Leishmania spp. using ELISA with a recombinant antigen (rTc24). *Mem. Inst. Oswaldo Cruz* **1997**, *92*, 791–793. [CrossRef] [PubMed]
8. Frank, F.M.; Fernandez, M.M.; Taranto, N.J.; Cajal, S.P.; Margni, R.A.; Castro, E.; Thomaz-Soccol, V.; Malchiodi, E.L. Characterization of human infection by Leishmania spp. in the Northwest of Argentina: Immune response, double infection with Trypanosoma cruzi and species of Leishmania involved. *Parasitology* **2003**, *126*, 31–39. [CrossRef]
9. Gil, J.; Cimino, R.; Lopez Quiroga, I.; Cajal, S.; Acosta, N.; Juarez, M.; Zacca, R.; Orellana, V.; Krolewiecki, A.; Diosque, P.; et al. [Reactivity of GST-SAPA antigen of Trypanosoma cruzi against sera from patients with Chagas disease and leishmaniasis]. *Medicina* **2011**, *71*, 113–119.
10. Wincker, P.; Bosseno, M.F.; Britto, C.; Yaksic, N.; Cardoso, M.A.; Morel, C.M.; Breniere, S.F. High correlation between Chagas' disease serology and PCR-based detection of Trypanosoma cruzi kinetoplast DNA in Bolivian children living in an endemic area. *FEMS Microbiol. Lett.* **1994**, *124*, 419–423. [CrossRef]
11. Castellano, L.R.; Filho, D.C.; Argiro, L.; Dessein, H.; Prata, A.; Dessein, A.; Rodrigues, V. Th1/Th2 immune responses are associated with active cutaneous leishmaniasis and clinical cure is associated with strong interferon-gamma production. *Hum. Immunol.* **2009**, *70*, 383–390. [CrossRef]
12. Rezende-Oliveira, K.; Sarmento, R.R.; Rodrigues, V., Jr. Production of cytokine and chemokines by human mononuclear cells and whole blood cells after infection with Trypanosoma cruzi. *Rev. Soc. Bras. Med. Trop.* **2012**, *45*, 45–50. [CrossRef] [PubMed]
13. Salhi, A.; Rodrigues, V., Jr.; Santoro, F.; Dessein, H.; Romano, A.; Castellano, L.R.; Sertorio, M.; Rafati, S.; Chevillard, C.; Prata, A.; et al. Immunological and genetic evidence for a crucial role of IL-10 in cutaneous lesions in humans infected with Leishmania braziliensis. *J. Immunol.* **2008**, *180*, 6139–6148. [CrossRef] [PubMed]
14. Campanelli, A.P.; Roselino, A.M.; Cavassani, K.A.; Pereira, M.S.; Mortara, R.A.; Brodskyn, C.I.; Goncalves, H.S.; Belkaid, Y.; Barral-Netto, M.; Barral, A.; et al. CD4+CD25+ T cells in skin lesions of patients with cutaneous leishmaniasis exhibit phenotypic and functional characteristics of natural regulatory T cells. *J. Infect. Dis.* **2006**, *193*, 1313–1322. [CrossRef] [PubMed]
15. de Araujo, F.F.; Correa-Oliveira, R.; Rocha, M.O.; Chaves, A.T.; Fiuza, J.A.; Fares, R.C.; Ferreira, K.S.; Nunes, M.C.; Keesen, T.S.; Damasio, M.P.; et al. Foxp3+CD25(high) CD4+ regulatory T cells from indeterminate patients with Chagas disease can suppress the effector cells and cytokines and reveal altered correlations with disease severity. *Immunobiology* **2012**, *217*, 768–777. [CrossRef] [PubMed]

16. Da-Cruz, A.M.; Bittar, R.; Mattos, M.; Oliveira-Neto, M.P.; Nogueira, R.; Pinho-Ribeiro, V.; Azeredo-Coutinho, R.B.; Coutinho, S.G. T-cell-mediated immune responses in patients with cutaneous or mucosal leishmaniasis: Long-term evaluation after therapy. *Clin. Diagn. Lab. Immunol.* **2002**, *9*, 251–256. [CrossRef] [PubMed]
17. Brelaz-de-Castro, M.C.; de Almeida, A.F.; de Oliveira, A.P.; de Assis-Souza, M.; da Rocha, L.F.; Pereira, V.R. Cellular immune response evaluation of cutaneous leishmaniasis patients cells stimulated with Leishmania (Viannia) braziliensis antigenic fractions before and after clinical cure. *Cell. Immunol.* **2012**, *279*, 180–186. [CrossRef] [PubMed]
18. Matos, G.I.; Covas Cde, J.; Bittar Rde, C.; Gomes-Silva, A.; Marques, F.; Maniero, V.C.; Amato, V.S.; Oliveira-Neto, M.P.; Mattos Mda, S.; Pirmez, C.; et al. IFNG +874T/A polymorphism is not associated with American tegumentary leishmaniasis susceptibility but can influence Leishmania induced IFN-gamma production. *BMC Infect. Dis.* **2007**, *7*, 33. [CrossRef]
19. Cabrera, M.; Shaw, M.A.; Sharples, C.; Williams, H.; Castes, M.; Convit, J.; Blackwell, J.M. Polymorphism in tumor necrosis factor genes associated with mucocutaneous leishmaniasis. *J. Exp. Med.* **1995**, *182*, 1259–1264. [CrossRef]
20. de Saldanha, R.R.; Martins-Papa, M.C.; Sampaio, R.N.; Muniz-Junqueira, M.I. Meglumine antimonate treatment enhances phagocytosis and TNF-alpha production by monocytes in human cutaneous leishmaniasis. *Trans. R. Soc. Trop. Med. Hyg.* **2012**, *106*, 596–603. [CrossRef]
21. Guedes, P.M.; Gutierrez, F.R.; Silva, G.K.; Dellalibera-Joviliano, R.; Rodrigues, G.J.; Bendhack, L.M.; Rassi, A., Jr.; Rassi, A.; Schmidt, A.; Maciel, B.C.; et al. Deficient regulatory T cell activity and low frequency of IL-17-producing T cells correlate with the extent of cardiomyopathy in human Chagas' disease. *PLoS Negl. Trop. Dis.* **2012**, *6*, e1630. [CrossRef]
22. Wanidworanun, C.; Strober, W. Predominant role of tumor necrosis factor-alpha in human monocyte IL-10 synthesis. *J. Immunol.* **1993**, *151*, 6853–6861. [PubMed]
23. Pissetti, C.W.; Correia, D.; de Oliveira, R.F.; Llaguno, M.M.; Balarin, M.A.; Silva-Grecco, R.L.; Rodrigues, V., Jr. Genetic and functional role of TNF-alpha in the development Trypanosoma cruzi infection. *PLoS Negl. Trop. Dis.* **2011**, *5*, e976. [CrossRef] [PubMed]
24. Reis, D.D.; Jones, E.M.; Tostes, S., Jr.; Lopes, E.R.; Gazzinelli, G.; Colley, D.G.; McCurley, T.L. Characterization of inflammatory infiltrates in chronic chagasic myocardial lesions: Presence of tumor necrosis factor-alpha+ cells and dominance of granzyme A+, CD8+ lymphocytes. *Am. J. Trop. Med. Hyg.* **1993**, *48*, 637–644. [CrossRef] [PubMed]
25. Rocha Rodrigues, D.B.; dos Reis, M.A.; Romano, A.; Pereira, S.A.; Teixeira Vde, P.; Tostes, S., Jr.; Rodrigues, V., Jr. In situ expression of regulatory cytokines by heart inflammatory cells in Chagas' disease patients with heart failure. *Clin. Dev. Immunol.* **2012**, *2012*, 361730. [CrossRef] [PubMed]
26. Sadeghian, G.; Ziaei, H.; Sadeghi, M. Electrocardiographic changes in patients with cutaneous leishmaniasis treated with systemic glucantime. *Ann. Acad. Med. Singap.* **2008**, *37*, 916–918.

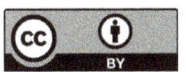

© 2020 by the authors. Licensee MDPI, Basel, Switzerland. This article is an open access article distributed under the terms and conditions of the Creative Commons Attribution (CC BY) license (http://creativecommons.org/licenses/by/4.0/).

MDPI
St. Alban-Anlage 66
4052 Basel
Switzerland
Tel. +41 61 683 77 34
Fax +41 61 302 89 18
www.mdpi.com

Tropical Medicine and Infectious Disease Editorial Office
E-mail: tropicalmed@mdpi.com
www.mdpi.com/journal/tropicalmed